Conduction Blockade
for
Postoperative
Analgesia

Conduction Blockade
for
Postoperative
Analgesia

Edited by

J. H. McClure BSc FCAnaes
Consultant Anaesthetist,
The Royal Infirmary, Edinburgh

and

J. A. W. Wildsmith MD FCAnaes
Consultant Anaesthetist,
The Royal Infirmary, Edinburgh

Edward Arnold
A division of Hodder & Stoughton
LONDON   MELBOURNE   AUCKLAND

© 1991 J. H. McClure and J. A. W. Wildsmith
First published in Great Britain 1991
British Library Cataloguing in Publication Data

Wildsmith, J. A.
  Conduction blockade for postoperative analgesia
  I. Tile   II. McClure, J. H.
  617.9

ISBN 0–340–55041–4

Typeset in 10/12 pt Palatino by Hewer Text Composition,
Edinburgh. Printed by St Edmundsbury Press Limited, Bury
St Edmunds, Suffolk, and bound by Hartnolls Ltd, Bodmin,
Cornwell for Edward Arnold, a publishing division of Hodder
and Stoughton Limited, Mill Road, Durton Green, Sevenoaks, Kent
TN13 2YA

Contents

Contributors

M. S. Brockway FCAnaes
Department of Anaesthetics, The Royal Infirmary, Edinburgh

K. Budd MB, ChB, FFARCS
Dept of Anaesthetics, The Royal Infirmary, Bradford

F. Cervero MB, ChB, PhD
Visceral Sensation Research Group, Department of Physiology, University of Bristol Medical School, Bristol

B. G. Covino PhD, MD
Dept of Anesthesia, Brigham and Women's Hospital, Harvard Medical School, Boston, Mass, USA

H. B. J. Fischer FFARCS
Department of Anaesthetics, The Alexandra Hospital, Redditch

R. G. Hill B.Pharm, PhD
Neuroscience Research Centre, Terlings Park, Harlow

A. Lee FCAnaes
Department of Anaesthetics, The Royal Infirmary, Edinburgh

J. M. A. Laird BSc, PhD
Neurobiology and Anesthesiology Branch, National institute of Health, NIDR, Bathesda, Maryland, USA.

J. H. McClure BSc, FCAnaes
Department Anaesthetics, The Royal Infirmary,
Edinburgh

M. Morgan FC Anaes,
Department of Anaesthetics, Hammersmith Hospital, Londony.

A. Mowbray BSc, MB, Ch.B, FFARCS
Department of Anaesthesia, Victoria Hospital, Kirkcaldy, Fife.

N. B. Scott FRCS, FC Anaes
Division of Anaesthesia, Royal Infirmary, Glasgow

B. E. Smith FFARCS
Department of Anaesthetics, Alexandra Hospital, Redditch

J. A. W. Wildsmith MD, FCAnaes
Department of Anaesthesia, The Royal Infirmary, Edinburgh

Foreword

Pain management as a central element in postoperative care has long been a focus for research endeavour. Sadly, surprisingly little of the results has been translated to practical help for the patient; the level of untreated pain after operations remains a scandal of modern medicine. Doctors John McClure and Tony Wildsmith have an outstanding record in the field of pain relief, and especially in the use of local anaesthetic techniques. Their concern is not just with research but in the teaching of trainees in anaesthesia, surgery and nursing. Their expertise is typified in the planning of this book and in the selection of those who have joined by contributing chapters. The result is a work which is both practical and authoritative. It will be of obvious value to anaesthetists and surgeons and I believe that the laboratory scientist and the nurse will find it a useful source, for unless all the disciplines work together for better pain relief the best solutions will elude us.

Professor Alastair A. Spence
May 1991

Preface

For the majority of patients, postoperative analgesia is provided by the intermittent intramuscular injection of an opioid, even though this is recognised as being a relatively ineffective method. Conceptually, the application of a drug close to a more peripheral part of the pain pathway for a discrete, potent action without complications is very attractive. This idea was conceived first by Alexander Wood in 1853, but it is only in the last two to three decades that significant advances towards successful utilisation of the principle have been made.

Two factors are probably relevant. First, increased use of local anaesthetic techniques (especially in obstetrics) has reminded anaesthetists of the benefits of analgesia without central depression. Secondly an explosion in knowledge of the physiology and pharmacology of the transmission of pain sensation has shown that drugs other than the local anaesthetics might be employed. The enthusiasm with which the spinal opioids were employed initially was a clear demonstration of the recognition of the need for such a technique. The spinal cord is far more than a simple relay station and many different types of drugs may have an action upon it.

Much of the recent research on pain has been at a very basic level and may seem divorced from the clinician dealing with patients in severe acute pain. The aim of this text is to bridge this gap and to indicate how drugs may be used to provide postoperative analgesia at the level of the spinal cord or peripheral nerve axon. For our purposes 'conduction blockade' is defined as pharmacological interruption of the pain pathway at the primary neurone or the synapse between it and the secondary neurone. The opening chapters describe the basic physiology of impulse transmission and indicate where and how different classes of drug may interrupt it. At the time of writing only the local anaesthetics, the opioids and the nonsteroidal agents have a clearly defined role in postoperative analgesia. However, current research indicates that many different classes of agent have an inhibitory action on pain transmission. Much of this research has been stimulated by concerns about chronic pain syndromes, but increasingly it seems that its immediate practical importance may well be in the management of acute pain. Awareness of how these agents work will enable the clinician to utilise them better if and when they become available.

Whatever the mechanism of drug action, the agent will need to reach its site of action; therefore knowledge of the factors that influence drug spread is essential. Ensuring that the drug reaches its target receptor is but one aspect of proper patient management, the nub of which is the provision of good quality analgesia while ensuring patient safety. Drug, technique and patient selection are thus all important. Properly managed these methods can make significant contributions to patient well being.

J. H. McClure

J. A. W. Wildsmith

Acknowledgements

We would like to thank our wives, Patricia and Fay, and our families for their continued support and forebearance of the time spent on the production of this book. Our thanks are also due to Mrs Cindy Middleton for her secretarial support, to Professor Spence for his foreword and to the individual authors for their contributions.

We would particularly like to acknowledge the support of Professor Ben Covino, whose original concept stimulated the project. His sudden and untimely death shortly before publication has been a great personal and professional loss.

1

Neurophysiology of postoperative pain

F. Cervero
J. M. A. Laird

Introduction

Surgical interventions cause, in the vast majority of cases, postoperative pain. Injury or damage to the skin and internal organs produces pain and most forms of surgery require the infliction of such injury. No matter how restricted the intervention or how well controlled the surgical procedure, surgery necessarily involves a certain amount of injury to the patient. Yet it is only recently that detailed consideration has been given to postoperative analgesia as an integral part of the surgical procedure. Much of this interest is due to the realization by surgeons and anaesthetists that postoperative analgesia not only improves the quality of life of the patient but also results in a faster recovery and hence reduced medical costs. All this represents a major departure from the medical view of pain prevalent in former times and is, to a large extent, the consequence of current social pressures. The contributions presented in this volume are good examples of the interest taken in postoperative analgesia and of the development of new methods for the prevention or relief of this form of pain.

Postoperative pain and analgesia are also of considerable interest to basic scientists studying the neurobiology of pain. Most of the current knowledge about the anatomy, physiology and pharmacology of nociceptive systems has been obtained from animal models of acute pain using experimental approaches involving the infliction of acute injury to animals under anaesthesia. This situation reproduces directly the circumstances of a surgical intervention, and therefore much of the information obtained from these experiments is of immediate relevance to clinicians interested in surgical and postoperative pain. Conversely, the clinical analysis of human postoperative pain provides the basic scientist with information on the sensory correlates of acute injury. This is of major importance for the interpretation of the results from animal experiments,

1

since such acute experiments under anaesthesia cannot obviously give any information about pain perception.

In this chapter the neural systems involved in the signalling and modulation of postoperative pain will be reviewed with reference to current knowledge of the basic mechanisms of acute pain. To this end, we will consider what is known about the signalling of acute injury by peripheral sensory receptors, the pathways transmitting this information to the central nervous system (CNS) and the reactions of spinal and supraspinal centres to these inputs from the periphery. The latter aspect is currently the subject of a good deal of scientific interest in relation to the changes induced in the CNS by an acute noxious stimulus such as that produced by a surgical intervention. Some of the treatments proposed for postoperative pain are directly aimed at preventing the increase in CNS excitability and alterations of neuronal properties that follow the arrival in the CNS of a nociceptive message.

Acute pain, injury pain and postoperative pain

All normal human beings can experience pain as the result of the application of noxious stimuli. Such stimuli are usually defined as those that produce injury, damage or potential damage to the skin, subcutaneous tissues or internal organs. In this context, pain is a normal sensory experience resulting from the excitation of peripheral sensory detectors which activate the appropriate spinal cord pathways and their sensory nuclei. Under these conditions the final perception of pain will depend on the interactions and modulations of the sensory message that take place at all relay stations within the CNS. This form of pain is *normal* pain and is part of the physiological sensory repertoire of all normal individuals (see Ref. 1 for a detailed discussion).[1]

Most forms of injury-induced pain begin with the activation of the system that mediates the perception of normal pain. Postoperative pain, which is the consequence of the injury produced by surgical intervention, is one such form of normal pain. In fact, it would be regarded as highly abnormal if a patient did not feel pain after a thoracotomy or after extensive abdominal surgery. Because it is usually short-lived and follows the time course of the recovery from the surgical intervention, postoperative pain is also a form of acute pain. In this sense, postoperative pain is part of the normal sensory response to an injury and is similar to the pain resulting from a skin burn or from any other kind of traumatic injury.

There are however, considerable variations in the relationship between injury and the perception of normal pain. It is well known that the levels of stress, attention and arousal of the subject can powerfully influence the intensity of the pain evoked by noxious peripheral stimuli. Postoperative pain can also vary in intensity and duration depending on the extent of the injury and on the kind of organ that has been the target of the surgical lesion.

All forms of injury to the skin and subcutaneous tissues are capable of evoking painful sensations. This is the reason for the consideration of injury-induced pain as part of a protective mechanism (*The psychical adjunct of a protective reflex:* Sherrington). The large number and variety of cutaneous nociceptors ensure that injuries to the skin are painful, well localized and capable of triggering protective reflexes such as withdrawal and flexion reflexes. Cutaneous nociceptors can also be sensitized by injury, thus contributing to the cutaneous hyperalgesia that develops after producing a skin lesion.

Injury to deep somatic structures such as muscles, ligaments and bones also evokes normal pain. This type of pain is duller than that evoked by cutaneous injury, and often takes the form of a persistent ache or cramp. In addition its localization is less precise than that of cutaneous pain. However, there is still a direct relationship between injury to deep somatic structures and the perception of normal pain.

In contrast with the pain produced by injury to somatic structures, pain of visceral origin is poorly localized and not directly related to the presence or extent of a lesion of internal organs. Extensive damage to the liver, the kidneys or the lungs does not provide any sensory feedback to the individual unless adjacent structures are also affected.[2] Normal visceral pain is usually evoked by stimuli that cause strong contractions of smooth muscle and/or ischaemia of the viscus. Thermal and mechanical injury of most internal organs is quite painless whereas minor forms of damage such as those produced by renal calculi are excruciatingly painful. It is not immediately clear why intense visceral pain should be evoked by situations that cannot be improved by natural therapies. It is even more puzzling that some life threatening stimuli, such as liver damage, are quite painless (see Ref. 3 for discussion). Because of this lack of correlation between injury and visceral pain, it has been proposed that a visceral noxious stimulus should be defined not as the stimulus that produces (or can produce) injury but as the stimulus that produces (or can produce) pain.[3]

It can, therefore, be concluded that postoperative pain is a normal pain sensation that forms part of the response of the individual to an acute surgical injury. The intensity, localization and nature of postoperative pain will depend, to a certain extent, on the organs affected by the surgical injury. Thus the magnitude of the lesion to somatic structures (skin, muscle, subcutaneous tissues) will determine the intensity and accurate localization of the pain. On the other hand, surgery involving internal organs can produce very variable forms of pain depending on the organs concerned and on the nature of the surgical intervention. For instance, abdominal surgery involving traction or manipulation of mesenteries or stretch of hollow organs can evoke much more intense visceral pain than surgery restricted to the liver or the lungs.

Signalling of injury

The skin, deep tissues and internal organs are innervated by a rich variety of sensory receptors which transmit information to the central nervous system about the modality, intensity and time course of external and internal stimuli. Among the many categories of sensory receptor there is a distinct group activated specifically by damaging or potentially damaging stimuli. Such sensory receptors are called nociceptors, a term that acknowledges the distinctiveness of these receptors in their being activated only by noxious stimuli.

Nociceptors are characterized by their ability to distinguish between noxious and innocuous events. This is a consequence of the two basic properties of nociceptors: (a) their high threshold for activation, that is, their lack of responsiveness to low intensity stimuli and (b) their capacity to encode noxious intensities of stimulation, that is, their stimulus-response functions are centred around noxious intensities of stimulation.

An injury such as that inflicted during a surgical intervention activates a variety of sensory receptors with both low and high thresholds. This complex stimulus results in a variety of diverse sensations dominated by the perception of postoperative pain. Whereas low threshold receptors may contribute to the blended and more complex forms of the postoperative sensation it is quite clear that information about the injury component of the surgical stimulus is encoded by nociceptors. In the following paragraphs the functional properties of cutaneous, deep and visceral nociceptors will be briefly reviewed. In addition, consideration will be given to the alterations in nociceptor sensitivity that follow the continuing presence of a lesion in the periphery and the development of the inflammatory process. These are intrinsic components of the healing process and are known to alter profoundly the properties of peripheral nociceptors.

Cutaneous nociceptors

The skin is innervated by two different kinds of nociceptors distinguished by the conduction velocity of their afferent fibres:

1. *A-δ nociceptors* These are connected to small myelinated fibres with conduction velocities between 5 and 30 m.s.$^{-1}$ and are sensitive, almost exclusively, to noxious mechanical stimuli.[4] They form free nerve endings in the superficial layers of the dermis with terminations that penetrate into the epidermis. Their response thresholds are much higher than those of the sensitive mechanoreceptors and their responses increase as the stimulus

intensity reaches damaging levels. These receptors respond particularly well to pinching or squeezing the skin or to a pin-prick.

2. *C nociceptors* These are connected to unmyelinated afferent fibres with conduction velocities of 1.5 m.s.$^{-1}$ or less. They are also part of the free nerve ending network of the skin and respond to noxious levels of mechanical thermal or chemical stimuli.[4, 5] In addition they are sensitive to many pain-producing substances such as bradykinin, capsaicin, potassium histamine, acetylcholine and strong acids. Because of their responses to several types of noxious stimuli, they are known as *polymodal* nociceptors.

If repeated noxious stimuli are applied to the skin, both A-δ and C nociceptors show a progressive lowering of their threshold for excitation, so that after repeated noxious stimuli they begin to respond to innocuous intensities of stimulation. This property, known as *sensitization* has been claimed to be responsible for the primary hyperalgesia that frequently accompanies skin injuries.[6] However, the secondary hyperalgesia, characterized by spontaneous pain or by pain evoked by innocuous stimulation around a zone of injury, depends also on excitability changes within the central nervous system.

Muscle and deep nociceptors

Specific nociceptors have also been described in deep tissues such as muscles, ligaments and joints. In muscles they are connected to A-δ afferent fibres (called Group III fibres in muscle nerves). Group III fibres respond to chemicals known to cause muscle pain, such as potassium ions, bradykinin or 5-HT, and to sustained contraction of the muscle.[7] Although they may have a role in muscle pain they seem best suited to act as *ergoreceptors*, that is sensors of muscle work for the purposes of cardiovascular adaptation to exercise. Group IV muscle fibres (unmyelinated afferent fibres) respond to noxious chemicals and to other noxious stimuli that produce muscle pain such as pressure or heat.[7] They are particularly sensitive to muscle contraction under ischaemia, a well known cause of intense muscle pain.

Joints are innervated by specific nociceptors which respond to noxious movements of the joint and are connected to afferent C fibres running in articular nerves.[8] Like muscle nociceptors, joint nociceptors are sensitive to a variety of pain-producing substances and can be sensitized by local inflammation of the joint.[8]

Visceral nociceptors

Visceral nociceptors have been described in the heart, lungs, respiratory tract, testes, biliary system, ureter and uterus.[3] Their common characteristic is to respond to stimuli known to cause visceral pain and only to levels of stimulation above the physiological range (Fig. 1.1). Such receptors are thought to be responsible for the signalling of events such as cardiac ischaemia, irritation of the airways, pulmonary congestion, lung embolism, testicular injury, biliary and renal colics or labour pain. Most of these receptors are connected to unmyelinated (C) afferent fibres.

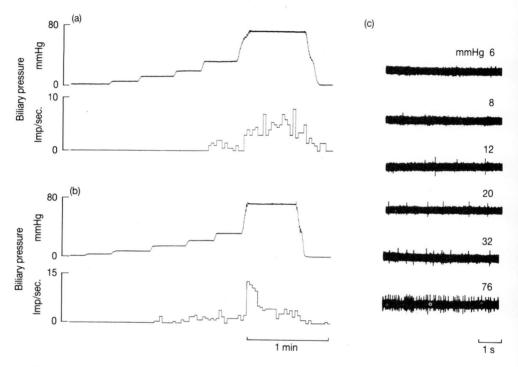

Figure 1.1   Visceral nociceptors from the biliary system of the ferret. The step changes in biliary pressure are displayed above the rate of firing of two single units from high threshold afferents (a and b). Samples of spike recordings at different biliary pressures are shown in c. b and c are from the same unit. (From reference 9).

Nociceptors and tissue damage

The vast majority of experimental studies of peripheral nociceptors have concentrated on the analysis of their responses to noxious stimulation of normal tissue. This kind of approach addresses only one aspect of the physiology of nociceptors: their capacity to signal the initial appearance of an injury or of potential damage. Over the last few years a number of new experimental models have been developed aimed at the study of the afferent innervation of injured tissue. These models address the question of possible changes in the response properties of nociceptive and non-nociceptive afferents due to the presence of an injury or lesion at peripheral level.

Two main findings have already emerged from these studies (a) nociceptors innervating damaged tissue are sensitized to the extent that they then respond to innocuous stimulation in that area. As mentioned earlier this represents the peripheral component of the mechanisms of hyperalgesia;[6] and (b) the presence of a persistent or sustained injury of the peripheral tissue brings into action sensory receptors previously unresponsive to low or high intensity mechanical stimuli.

The second observation is particularly intriguing as it means that certain organs of the body contain sensory receptors that respond only under physiopathological conditions once the organ has sustained an injury. This category of sensory receptor has been described in inflamed joints,[8] hypoxic ureter[10] and inflamed viscera such as the bladder and colon.[11] If this represents a general category of sensory receptor then it could be that conditions such as postoperative pain might be due to the activation of sensory channels previously unresponsive or inactive. It would also mean that prevention of sustained injury and of tissue inflammation could help to reduce postoperative pain.

Peripheral pathways and nerve fibres involved in the signalling of acute injury

The afferent fibres that transmit injury-related information to the CNS are among the slowest and thinnest of all nerve fibres. The majority of somatic nociceptors are connected to unmyelinated (C) afferent fibres and only a minority of nociceptors are connected to small myelinated (A-δ) afferents. In the case of the innervation of internal organs, the vast majority of visceral afferent fibres (over 90 per cent) are also unmyelinated with less than 10 per cent being small myelinated.

The two types of cutaneous nociceptive afferent that innervate the skin (A-δ and C) are supposed to mediate acute pain of different qualities. A brief noxious stimulus applied to the skin results in an early pricking pain (first pain) and a late burning sensation (second pain).[12] The analysis of the latency of first and second pain, and the observation that the two sensations cannot be separated when the stimulus is applied to the head or shoulders, supports the hypothesis that the first pain is mediated by nociceptors connected to A-δ fibres and the second pain results from the excitation of C-fibre nociceptors. Microneurographic studies of human nerves have supported this proposal by showing that microstimulation of A-δ nociceptors evokes pricking pain whereas stimulation of C-fibre nociceptors evokes pain of a burning quality.[13–15] In all cases, microstimulation of single afferent fibres results in sensations referred to the receptive field of the receptor under study.

The nociceptive afferent innervation of the skin and other somatic structures (muscles, ligaments, joints) is mediated by nerve fibres coursing in somatic nerves. These are primary afferent fibres whose cell bodies are all located in the dorsal root ganglia and, in the case of the innervation of the face, in the trigeminal ganglion. The central branches of these afferent fibres enter the spinal cord or the trigeminal spinal nucleus where they make contact with second-order neurones at the origin of spinal sensory tracts.

The nociceptive afferent innervation of viscera is also mediated by primary afferent fibres. Some of these afferent fibres run in parasympathetic nerves, such as the vagus and pelvic nerves, and have their cell bodies in the corresponding cranial and sacral sensory ganglia. Other visceral afferents join sympathetic nerves and reach the spinal nerves via the *rami comunicantes*.

Clinical studies using a combination of stimulation and blocking techniques have repeatedly shown that many forms of abdominal pain are evoked by stimulation of sympathetic, but not parasympathetic nerves, and are relieved by section or blockade of sympathetic, but not parasympathetic nerve trunks.[16] Therefore, it would appear that many forms of visceral pain are signalled by afferent fibres in sympathetic nerves and that the afferent innervation mediated by parasympathetic nerves is largely concerned with regulatory, but not sensory, aspects of gut physiology.

Peripheral distribution of visceral nociceptive fibres

Visceral primary afferent fibres projecting to the CNS via sympathetic nerves have their cell bodies in thoraco-lumbar spinal ganglia and their central projections enter the spinal cord at levels between T_{2-3} and L_{2-3}.

It has been known for some time that the total number of primary afferent fibres involved in the transmission of visceral nociceptive information is quite small. Recent studies, using neuronal tracing and labelling methods, have established that visceral afferent fibres constitute less than 10 per cent of the total afferent inflow to the thoraco-lumbar spinal cord.[17] This low density of innervation is particularly striking when taking into account the large surface area of the gastrointestinal tract, and is probably the reason for the diffuse nature of gastrointestinal pain. It must be noted that this region of the spinal cord receives its somatic input from the body areas with the poorest sensory discrimination (i.e. the back and the abdomen), whereas the visceral input to the thoraco-lumbar cord mediates pain from all upper abdominal organs including the stomach, the duodenum, the biliary tract, the pancreas and the small intestine. Yet the former sensations require 90 per cent or more of the total afferent input to the spinal cord whereas all visceral pain from the upper abdomen is mediated by less than 10 per cent of all spinal afferents.

Internal organs therefore have an extremely low density of sensory innervation, particularly by those afferent fibres that mediate the sensations of visceral pain. This explains why some viscera, such as gut, appear to be insensitive or require considerable stimulation before giving rise to pain. One such form of stimulation is the intense and persistent contraction of the intestinal wall that evokes colic pain. These contractions activate maximally and simultaneously the few nociceptive afferent fibres present in a given loop of intestine, and in this way evoke painful sensations in synchrony with the motor events. Smaller, irregular or less persistent contractions are probably insufficient to excite enough afferents with the intensity or synchrony necessary to activate nociceptive pathways in the central nervous system.

Efferent functions of nociceptive afferent fibres

It has been known for some time that an intact innervation is required for the maintenance of an adequate trophism of target organs and for the normal operation of the processes of tissue healing and repair. It is a common clinical observation that the interruption of the normal nerve supply to the skin or to internal organs induces trophic alterations of the peripheral tissue which include a very poor response to injury (i.e. the peripheral dysfunctions associated with diabetic neuropathies or the presence of persistent cutaneous ulcers in denervated skin).

Many of the trophic functions attributed to the innervation of peripheral tissue are currently interpreted in terms of the so-called *axon reflex*. Lewis proposed that collateral branches of nociceptive afferents had an efferent function in the skin.[18] This function is expressed by cutaneous vasodilatation and by increases in capillary permeability evoked by the release of active compounds from these collateral branches of nociceptive afferents following the activation of the nociceptive ending. According to this proposal a nociceptive afferent fibre can have a dual afferent–efferent role: the signalling of peripheral injury by the nociceptive sensory ending and the initiation of local defence reactions by the effector ending.

There is a considerable amount of experimental evidence supporting the concept of a dual role of nociceptive cutaneous afferents.[19] However, current thinking has eliminated the need for a separate collateral branch as the effector in the *axon reflex*, since it is now thought to be possible for the vasoactive compounds to be released by the same endings that contain the sensory receptor mechanism (Fig. 1.2).

The substances known to be released following the activation of cutaneous nociceptive afferents include substance P, histamine, bradykinin, prostaglandins and leukotrienes. Some are released directly by the afferent fibre endings whereas others (such as histamine and the prostaglandins) can be released by the subsequent excitation of mast cells. The combined effect of these compounds is a local vasodilatation and an increase in capillary permeability which help the movement of blood constituents into the interstitial space of the injured tissue. This initiates the inflammatory response which is the very first step in the process of tissue defence and repair.

In addition to their vasoactive properties, many of the substances released by nociceptive afferents following tissue injury are also known to alter the properties of the nociceptors themselves.[19] This leads to sensitization of nociceptive endings and – according to recent evidence[8] – to the coming into action of previously *silent* nociceptors.

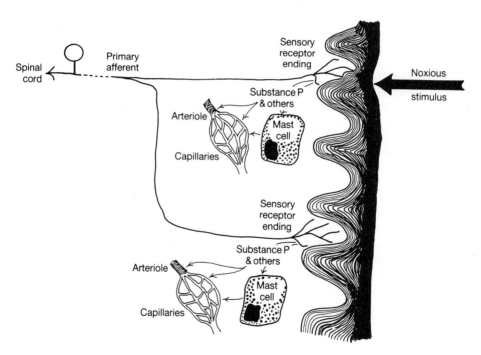

Figure 1.2 Diagram to show the proposed dual receptor-effector role for nociceptive cutaneous afferents. Stimulation of a nociceptor (top) leads to impulses travelling along the primary afferent fibre towards the spinal cord. The sensory receptor ending releases vasoactive compounds into the surrounding tissue. Impulses also travel back towards the skin along collateral branches of the afferent fibre and excite other sensory receptor endings. (bottom), which also release vasoactive compounds.

Thus, the presence of a peripheral injury such as that induced by a surgical intervention is initially signalled by nociceptive endings which in turn trigger a number of local and general reactions. First, nociceptive information is transmitted to the spinal cord and the brain and this leads to the perception of the injury-induced pain. Subsequent to their activation, nociceptive endings release a number of chemicals which initiate a local inflammation of the injured area. Finally, the active substances released in the inflamed tissue contribute to changes in the excitability of peripheral nociceptors which result in sensitization of the receptor endings. This leads to hyperalgesia of the injured area and can contribute to the secondary hyperalgesia often observed in regions close to the injury, but not actually affected by it.[6]

From the point of view of the prevention of postoperative pain, it is clear that suppressing peripheral nociceptive signals by local anaesthetics will also reduce the intensity of the sensitization of peripheral nociceptors and thus help to alleviate the hyperalgesia of the injured region during the postoperative recovery. Of course, eliminating the nociceptive afferent response will also interfere with the triggering of the local inflammatory reaction and can therefore reduce its beneficial effects. A better procedure would be to develop drugs that could eliminate the actions of the chemicals responsible for the sensitization of nociceptors – and hence the local hyperalgesia – but would preserve the vasoactive properties of these compounds and therefore the initiation of the inflammatory reaction.

Spinal mechanisms of pain and their reactions to acute injury

It is clear from the preceding pages that peripheral mechanisms can make an important contribution to the sensation produced by acute injury. The activation of peripheral receptors connected to primary afferents is the means by which events in the periphery are signalled, hence changes in their properties, such as the sensitization produced by acute injury, will alter the message arriving at the CNS. However, the activity of nociceptive primary afferents is not necessarily directly related to the painful sensation evoked by a noxious stimulus,[20] and similarly the changes in responses of peripheral receptors to damage cannot explain all of the features of the painful sensation evoked by an acute injury, thus, as might be expected, the processing of afferent input by the CNS is also important.

The primary afferent fibres innervating the nociceptors in the periphery have cell bodies in the dorsal root ganglia, enter the spinal cord via the dorsal roots and terminate within the dorsal horn of the spinal grey matter. Dorsal horn neurones receiving this input are the first point at which integration of these signals occurs. They also receive inputs both from higher centres and from other spinal neurones, and thus provide the first opportunity for descending and intraspinal modulation of the nociceptive message. The spinal cord is not just a relay station; dorsal horn neurones perform substantial amounts of processing of the afferent input. Hence there is currently a good deal of interest in the effects of acute injury on the spinal mechanisms responsible for the initial integration and modulation of noxious input. Evidence is now accumulating that spinal neurones can also become *sensitized* by noxious stimuli, and thus contribute to the sensations associated with tissue injury or inflammation.

The first part of this section will describe briefly the organization of the primary afferent input into the spinal cord and the characteristics of nociceptive dorsal horn neurones. We will then consider the way in which spinal systems react to acute injury, such as that produced by a surgical intervention, as compared to minor noxious stimulation or chronic and neuropathic pain states.

Termination of nociceptive afferents within the spinal cord

The intracellular labelling of single, functionally identified primary afferent fibres has provided unequivocal evidence as to the sites and modes of termination of afferents within the spinal cord. It seems that the termination site of primary afferents is determined largely by the functional properties of the receptor ending and the peripheral target innervated.

Large myelinated (A-β) fibres connected to low threshold cutaneous mechanoreceptors terminate in some or all of laminae* III, IV, V and the dorsal part of lamina VI. There is essentially no input from these axons to laminae I or II.[22] Similarly, low threshold cutaneous mechanoreceptors with fine myelinated (A-δ) afferent fibres terminate in lamina III and its border with lamina II.[23]

Nociceptors in general have unmyelinated or fine myelinated axons. Cutaneous high threshold mechanoreceptors with A-δ axons terminate in lamina I, and most have branches terminating in lamina V. Some also have terminals in the mid-line and contralaterally in laminae I and V. Cutaneous nociceptors with unmyelinated (C) fibres terminate predominantly in lamina II, although some also have terminals in laminae I and/or III-IV.[24] Nociceptive afferents from deep tissues (muscle and joints) terminate in laminae I, C, V–VI and the dorsal layers of lamina VII. There are no projections to laminae II, III or IV from deep tissue.[25, 26] Fine

---

* The spinal grey matter has been divided into ten layers or laminae on anatomical grounds. The dorsal horn corresponds to laminae I to VI (dorsal to ventral).[21]

afferents from viscera project to lamina I and bilaterally to laminae V and X (Fig. 1.3)[27, 28] Some unmyelinated visceral afferents also have a few collaterals in lamina II, but this lamina seems to be mostly concerned with the processing of input from skin nociceptors with unmyelinated afferent fibres.

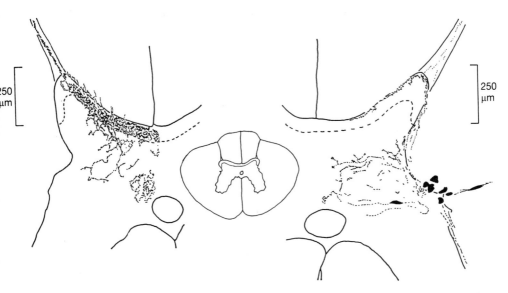

Figure 1.3 Reconstruction from 3 (left) and seven (right) 80 μm transverse serial sections of the projections of somatic (left) and visceral (right) afferent fibres to the T_9 segment of the spinal chord of the cat. Note the absence of a visceral afferent projection to the substantia gelantinosa (lamina II) whose ventral border is indicated by the dotted line. (Modified from reference 29).

Spinal neurochemistry and acute injury

The development of powerful immunohistochemical techniques for the detection of biologically active compounds in nerve cells has resulted in the discovery of a large number of peptides and other substances in primary afferent neurones and in spinal cord second-order cells. Substances detected in primary afferent fibres, presumed to include nociceptive afferents, include: substance P, Cholecystokinin (CCK), Vasoactive Intestinal Peptide (VIP), Fluoride Resistant Acid Phosphatase (FRAP), Calcitonin Gene Related Peptide (CGRP), Enkephalin (ENK) and Dynorphin (DYN). Many of these compounds (and quite a few others) are also found in second-order spinal cord neurones, including those at the origin of ascending somatosensory pathways.[30]

The discovery of this plethora of potential transmitters has fuelled speculation as to their functional role. Models of organization of the first nociceptive relay in the dorsal horn have been postulated on the basis of the putative transmitters that mediate the transmission of injury-related information, with substance P playing a key role in this relay.[31] The possible roles of endogenous opioids in the modulation of nociceptive information in the spinal cord have also been the object of considerable speculation. To date the experimental evidence for any of these compounds being classical neurotransmitters is tenuous and therefore their putative roles are usually discussed in terms of their actions as *neuromodulators*. This is a somewhat imprecise label which in many cases is meant to hide our ignorance as to what the functions of these compounds are.

However, immunohistochemical techniques have proved to be very useful as labels for groups of primary afferents or of cells, thus enabling the examination of their anatomical distribution within the spinal cord. These procedures permit – often in combination with standard neuroanatomical tracing techniques – the marking of identified afferents and cells and their subsequent morphological and ultrastructural study. The application of immunohistochemistry to the study of spinal cord circuitry has provided a good deal of information about the cones of projection within the grey matter of identified groups of primary afferents.[32]

In addition, there are a number of studies of the changes in the levels and distribution of putative *neuromodulators* in spinal neurones following peripheral injury. For instance the levels of the opioid peptide, Dynorphin increase in the dorsal horn after the induction of experimental inflammation of a limb.[33] Conversely, the number of opioid receptors in the superficial dorsal horn of the spinal cord decreases when peripheral nerves are cut.[34] The experimental induction of a peripheral neuropathy also results in the decrease of some primary afferent peptides (substance P, CGRP) and in the increase of Dynorphin levels in spinal cord neurones.[35] Although the functional significance of these findings is obscure it is nevertheless relevant to the present discussion to point out that the neurochemistry of the spinal nociceptive relay can change as a consequence of a peripheral injury such as those commonly inflicted by surgical interventions.

Nociceptive neurones in the dorsal horn of the spinal cord

Nociceptive dorsal horn neurones are concentrated in laminae I–II and IV–VI, corresponding with the regions in which the nociceptive afferents terminate. These neurones can be divided into two groups on the basis of their cutaneous afferent input (see Fig. 1.4); (a) neurones with inputs from both low threshold afferents and from nociceptive afferents (multireceptive or Class 2 neurones), and (b) neurones with an exclusive input from nociceptive afferents (nocireceptive or Class 3 neurones). Nociceptive visceral

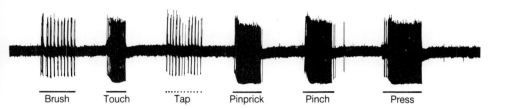

Brush   Touch   Tap   Pinprick   Pinch   Press

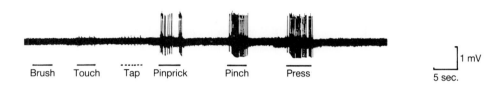

Brush   Touch   Tap   Pinprick   Pinch   Press

1 mV

5 sec.

Figure 1.4 Oscilloscope traces showing the response of two different dorsal horn neurones in the spinal cord of a rat to natural stimulation of their cutaneous receptive fields. The upper trace shows a Class 2 neurone responding to both innocuous and noxious stimulation. The lower trace shows a Class 3 neurone responding to noxious stimuli only.

and deep inputs to the spinal cord are processed by nociceptive dorsal horn neurones which also have cutaneous input; there is no *private pathway* for information from these tissues.

Class 2 neurones Some Class 2 neurones are found in laminae I–II, but the majority are located in the deep dorsal horn, and both groups include neurones which project to supraspinal centres. They generally receive a very convergent input from a wide variety of different primary afferent types and a fairly large skin area. These cells are not obvious candidates for a role in distinguishing a noxious from an innocuous stimulus, or in the precise localization of a stimulus, although various mechanisms by which such information may be extracted from their responses have been proposed.[36] However, Class 2 cells may well have an important role in encoding the intensity of stimuli and integration and modulation dependent on the immediate past history of the organism.

Class 3 neurones The highest concentration of Class 3 cells is in the superficial layer of the dorsal horn, although some are also found in the deeper laminae. Some have axons which project rostrally to terminate in the mid-brain and thalamus. Since these cells respond only to noxious stimuli they may have a role in distinguishing noxious from innocuous events. Class 3 neurones have small receptive fields, and are thus well suited to convey precise information about the location of a noxious stimulus on the body surface.

The effect of acute injury on dorsal horn neurones

The way in which spinal systems processing noxious stimuli react to acute injury is perhaps best considered as part of the whole scope of responses of the system to inputs ranging from minor noxious stimuli to chronic and neuropathic pain states. The range of responses can be described in terms of three components, as follows:

Phase 1   The response of the system to noxious, but non-damaging stimuli, such as the minor knocks that are sustained during the course of everyday life. If such a stimulus is sufficiently intense or prolonged,

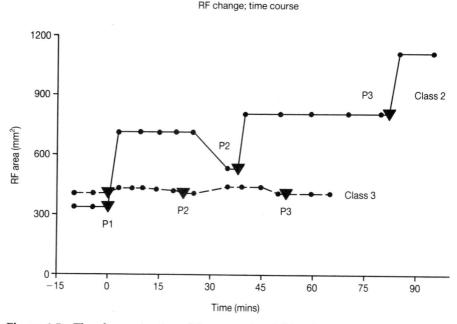

Figure 1.5   The change in size of the receptive fields of one Class 2 neurone and one Class 3 neurone, both recorded in barbiturate anaesthetised rates, over time during a series of noxious pinches. The application of three pinch stimuli (P1, P2 and P3) are indicated by closed inverted triangles. Measurements of the receptive field area between pinches are indicated by small circles. (From reference 38).

substantial increases in the excitability of the Class 2 neurones (but not the Class 3 neurones) may be seen. Examples of this include the increasing responses to C-fibre strength electrical stimulation known as wind-up,[37] or large increases in receptive field size[38] (Fig. 1.5). If the stimulus is not repeated and no injury is sustained, the effects are short-lived and local.

Phase 2   The response of the system to repeated, sustained or damaging stimuli such as the acute injury produced by a surgical intervention. The afferent input to the dorsal horn neurones under these conditions will be from sensitized peripheral receptors as described earlier and therefore changed, but in addition, the evidence would suggest that both the Class 2 and Class 3 nociceptive systems may alter their response properties.

Class 2 neurones seem to be very easily induced to change by relatively minor noxious stimuli; thus more severe stimuli are likely to enhance and sustain such changes. Class 3 neurones are more resistant to change, but increased excitability, expressed as increases in receptive field size and greater spontaneous and evoked firing, has been observed in Class 3 neurones after skin burns,[39] local inflammation[40, 41] and noxious chemical stimulation of the skin[42, 43] or deep tissues.[44] The onset of these changes in the responses of the Class 3 neurones has a long time course in many cases; 6–8 hours after the induction of a local inflammation for example.[40] Interestingly, noxious stimulation of deep tissues seems to be more effective in producing these changes than skin stimulation.[45, 44]

The sustained increase in excitability of the spinal cord systems responsible for processing noxious input induced by the acute injury of a surgical intervention may well make a significant contribution to postoperative painful sensation. This supposition is supported by the effectiveness of the clinical use of spinal blocks during surgery.

These changes can be regarded as a property of the *normal* CNS, just as the pain associated with surgical interventions is normal pain. Past events and current circumstances are taken into account in the processing of new inputs, but the system remains in equilibrium over the long term.

Phase 3   The response of the system to very prolonged and severe noxious inputs or to damage to the nervous system. Chronic conditions such as arthritis or nerve injuries produce qualitative changes in spinal cord systems, such as changes in the properties and proportions of dorsal horn neuronal populations,[46] and the formation of new anatomical connections between neurones.[47]

These conditions are associated with abnormal pain sensation, and probably represent an *abnormal* CNS resulting from the absence of a section of the normal input, or an excessively intense and/or prolonged input. In this case, the equilibrium has been pushed to a new set-point, and a qualitative change of the system produced. This third response of spinal cord pain mechanisms is unlikely to be encountered as a result of uncomplicated surgical intervention, except in cases in which peripheral nerves are sectioned or damaged.

It would seem that interrupting the noxious input produced by a surgical intervention using peripheral or spinal blocks will help to prevent the development of the kind of changes in spinal systems that characterize *phase 2*, and therefore will contribute to the prevention or lessening of postoperative pain. However, if the system moves outside the normal range towards an abnormal state (*phase 3*), procedures aimed at the periphery alone are unlikely to affect the outcome.

Contribution of descending influences to the reaction of spinal systems to acute injury

Descending influences arising from supraspinal centres are clearly very important to the proper functioning of the spinal cord in humans, since the interruption of such inputs by section of the spinal cord produces a complete cessation of activity in spinal systems for a prolonged period (spinal shock). The spinal cord systems that process noxious inputs are known to be subject to supraspinal influences. Thus higher brain centres modulate the input into the system at the first available point. This modulation can have two opposite actions; either to inhibit or to enhance the transmission of the nociceptive message. The circumstances of the individual will determine which of these two mechanisms is the more important in the final perception of the painful sensation.

Descending inhibition of spinal systems

The reduction or total abolition of a painful sensation occurs under some natural circumstances in which there is no medical or surgical intervention. The two principal examples of this *endogenous* modulation of a painful sensation are that it can be inhibited (a) by a more intense pain sensation from another part of the body, and (b) in circumstances of acute stress and/or arousal.

There is now a good deal of evidence for a descending control system that could provide the neural substrate for the observation that *pain inhibits pain*. It has been shown that a noxious stimulus applied to one part of the body will inhibit the activity of nociceptive neurones in the spinal cord whose receptive fields lie outside that body area. This system is termed *Diffuse Noxious Inhibitory Controls* (DNIC) because of its widespread, non-somatotopic effects.[48] Class 2 neurones in particular are affected by DNIC. The strength of the inhibitory effect depends on the intensity of the conditioning stimulus; a strong noxious stimulus produces greater inhibition than a weak one. The mechanism that mediates DNIC must include a supraspinal component, since this type of inhibitory effect is much reduced after spinalization.

There is also a large body of literature showing that the responses of nociceptive spinal cord neurones can be inhibited by the stimulation of various supraspinal structures.[49, 50] Similarly, stimulation of brainstem areas, in particular the periaquaductal grey matter of the mid-brain (PAG), in awake animals can evoke *stimulation-produced analgesia* or a state in which severe noxious stimuli produce no external signs of discomfort.[51] Another form of descending inhibition acting on nociceptive dorsal horn neurones is *tonic descending inhibition*, which is revealed as increased excitability when descending supraspinal messages are interrupted by spinalization.[52] The supraspinal sources of tonic descending inhibition do not seem to coincide with all the sites from which stimulation-produced analgesia can be evoked, so the two types may be manifestations of separate systems. These types of descending inhibition may form the neural basis of the analgesia produced by stressful situations. However, these various forms of descending inhibition are not necessarily very selective for noxious input, and may represent a generalized inhibition of inputs to the somatosensory system.[51, 52]

Descending inhibition of the responses of dorsal horn neurones is likely to be evoked by the noxious stimulation of a surgical intervention; in particular, it has been suggested that tonic descending inhibition of spinal systems seen in experimental animals is activated by the trauma of surgery.[53]

Descending excitation of spinal systems

Enhancement of the nociceptive message may be mediated in part by descending excitation of spinal cord neurones. It has been demonstrated that some nociceptive neurones in the spinal cord are excited by stimulation of brainstem sites, and there are also several reports of spinal nociceptive neurones under tonic descending excitation from supraspinal systems.[3] This excitation may reflect the higher degree of excitability and arousal that generally accompanies a painful experience. Alternatively it has been proposed that this type of descending excitation will enhance the activity of sensory neurones sufficiently to generate a spinal-bulbo-spinal positive feedback loop.[54] Such a loop would maintain central activity beyond the application of the stimulus, and also perhaps account for the spread of a painful sensation beyond the original area of injury (Fig. 1.6).

It seems likely that although the stress and trauma of surgery will activate descending inhibitory mechanisms, as part of the arousal mechanism the descending excitation of sensory pathways enhancing somatosensory awareness may well also be important in the perception of postoperative pain. Preventing the arrival of nociceptive messages to the spinal cord

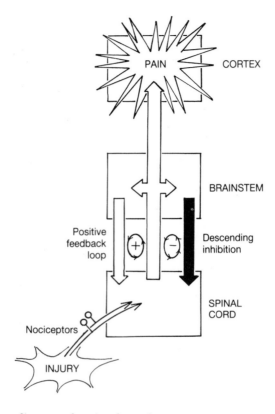

Figure 1.6   Box diagram showing how the nociceptive message that results from a peripheral injury may both be enhanced by a positive feedback loop between the spinal cord and brainstem and suppressed by descending inhibition.

during a surgical intervention by a peripheral or spinal block will therefore prevent the triggering of the positive feedback reactions that lead to prolonged postoperative pain.

Summary and conclusions

1.   Post operative pain is the natural consequence of the injury caused by a surgical intervention. It is normally due to the activation of the nociceptive system that mediates the perception of injury-related pain and, as such, it is a normal response of the body to surgical trauma to peripheral tissues. Because of the differences in sensory innervation between somatic and visceral structures and between different viscera, the intensity, localization and nature of postoperative pain depend on the organs affected by the surgical injury.

2. Acute injury is signalled by the activation of peripheral nociceptors. There is a substantial body of evidence for the existence of specific nociceptors in the skin and other somatic tissues. There is also some evidence for the presence of specific nociceptors in viscera although these probably co-exist with non-specific receptors and with sensory receptors activated only after the occurrence of tissue damage. All nociceptors can be sensitized by injury so that their thresholds for activation become lower thus contributing to the mechanisms of hyperalgesia.

3. The density of sensory innervation of internal organs is considerably lower than that of the skin and other somatic tissues. This explains why some viscera appear to be insensitive or require considerable stimulation before giving rise to an ill-localized and dull pain.

4. The presence of a peripheral injury activates peripheral nociceptors which in turn trigger a number of local reactions by the release of certain chemicals that initiate a local inflammation of the injured area. These substances can also alter the sensitivity of the peripheral receptors leading to hyperalgesia and increased pain sensitivity of the zone lesioned.

5. Nociceptive afferents from the periphery terminate in the dorsal horn of the spinal grey matter, predominantly in laminae I–II and IV–VI. Dorsal horn neurones perform a considerable amount of processing of this afferent input, and the spinal relay is also important as the first point at which modulation by descending inputs from supraspinal centres occurs. There are two types of nociceptive dorsal horn neurones; Class 3 neurones, which receive input exclusively from nociceptive afferents, and are thought to have a sensory-discriminative role, and Class 2 neurones, which receive both nociceptive and innocuous inputs, and are thought to play a role in modulation and integration of responses to noxious inputs.

6. The response of the spinal cord systems to a noxious input can be considered as three phases. Minor noxious stimuli can produce changes in Class 2 cell response properties, but Class 3 cells are less affected. Acute injuries induce changes in both systems, which may contribute to the characteristics of the painful sensations associated with these injuries. Very prolonged severe input or damage to the nervous system produce more permanent changes in the CNS, which may result in abnormal pain sensation.

7. Descending inputs from supraspinal structures, inhibitory or excitatory, are important in the spinal processing of noxious stimuli. Inhibitory mechanisms contribute to the analgesia produced by stressful situations, and the inhibition of one painful sensation by another. Excitatory mechanisms, including the proposed bulbospinal positive feedback loop, may well contribute to the sustaining of painful sensations beyond the duration of stimulus initiating the reaction.

8. The prevention and treatment of postoperative pain requires an approach that takes into account both the peripheral and the central

neurophysiological mechanisms. It is clear that preventing the injury-induced responses from reaching the central nervous system will also prevent the triggering of central reactions that sustain and enhance postoperative pain.

References

1. Cervero F. Neurophysiological aspects of pain and pain therapy. In *The Therapy of Pain* Swerdlow, M. (ed.) Lancaster: MTP Press, 1986: 1–30.
2. Mackenzie, J. *Symptoms and Their Interpretation*. Shaw. London: 1909.
3. Cervero, F. Visceral Pain. In: *Proceedings of the Vth World Congress on Pain*. Dubner R., Gebhart G. F. & Bond M. R. (eds) Amsterdam: Elsevier 1988: 216–26
4. Burgess P. R. & Perl E. R. Cutaneous mechanoreceptors and nociceptors. In: *Somatosensory System, Handbook of Sensory Physiology, Vol 11* Iggo, A. (ed.) Heidelberg, Springer: 1973: 29–78.
5. Beck P. W., Handwerker H. O. & Zimmermann M. Nervous outflow from the cat's foot during noxious radiant heat stimulation. *Brain Res.* 1974; **67**: 373–86.
6. Meyer R. A., Campbell J. N. & Raja S. N. Peripheral neural mechanisms of cutaneous hyperalgesia. *Adv. Pain Res. Ther.* 1985 **9**: 53–71.
7. Mense S. & Schmidt R. F. Muscle pain: which receptors are responsible for the transmission of noxious stimuli. In: *Physiological Aspects of Clinical Neurology*, Rose, J. E. (ed.) Oxford: Blackwell, 1977: 265–278.
8. Schaible H. G. & Schmidt R. F. Direct observations of the sensitization of articular afferents during an experimental arthritis. In: *Proceedings of the Vth World Congress on Pain*. Dubner R., Gebhart G. F. & Bond M. R. (eds) Amsterdam: Elsevier, 1988: 44–50.
9. Cervero F. Afferent activity evoked by natural stimulation of the biliary system in the ferret *Pain* 1982 **13**: 137–51.
10. Cervero F. & Sann, H. Mechanically evoked responses of afferent fibres innervating the guinea-pig's ureter: an *in vitro* study. *J. Physiol.* 1989; **412**: 245–66
11. Habler H.-J., Janig W. & Koltzenburg M. A novel type of unmyelinated chemosensitive nociceptor in the acutely inflamed urinary bladder. *Agents and Actions* 1988 **25**: 219–21.
12. Collins W. F. Jr, Nulsen F. E. & Randt C. T. Relation of peripheral nerve fibre size and sensation in man. *Arch. Neurol. Chicago. 1960* **3**: 381–5.
13. Torebjörk H. E. Nociceptor activation and pain. *Phil. Trans. R. Soc. Lond. B.* 1985 **308**: 227–34.
14. Torebjörk H. E., Valbo, A. B. & Ochoa, J. L. Intraneural microstimulation in man. Its relation to specificity of tactile sensations. *Brain* 1987 **110**: 1497–508.
15. Ochoa J. L. & Torebjörk H. E. Sensations evoked by intraneural microstimulation of C nociceptor fibres in human skin nerves. *J. Physiol.* 1989 **415**: 583–600
16. White J. C. Sensory innervation of the viscera. Studies on visceral afferent neurones in man based on neurosurgical procedures for the

relief of intractable pain. *Res. Pub. Assoc. Res. Nerv. Ment. Dis.* 1943 **23**: 373–90

17. Cervero F., Connell L. A. & Lawson S. N. Somatic and visceral primary afferants in the lower thoracic dorsal root ganglia of the cat. *J. Comp. Neurol.* 1984; **412**: 245–66.
18. Lewis T. *Pain*. London: Macmillan, 1942.
19. Lisney S. J. W. & Bharali L. A. M. The axon reflex: an out-dated idea or a valid hypothesis? *N. I. P. S.* 1989 **4**: 45–8
20. Adriansen H., Gybels J., Handwerker H. O. & Van Hees J. Nociceptor discharges and sensations due to prolonged noxious stimulation – a paradox. *Human Neurobiol.* 1984; **3**: 53–8
21. Rexe B. (1984). A cytoarchitectonic atlas of the spinal cord in the cat. *J. Comp. Neurol.* 1984 **96**: 415–66.
22. Brown A. G. The dorsal horn of the spinal cord. *Q. J. Exp. Physiol.* 1982; **67**: 193–212.
23. Light A. R. & Perl E. R. Spinal termination of functiuonally identified primary afferent neurons with slowly conducting myelinated fibres. *J. Comp. Neurol.* 1979 **186**: 135–50.
24. Sugiura Y., Lee C. L. & Perl E. R. Central projections of identified unmyelinated (C) afferent fibres innervating mammallan skin. *Science* 1986 **234**: 358–361.
25. Mense S. Slowly conducting afferent fibres from deep tissues: neuro- biological properties and central nervous actions. *Progr. Sensory Physiol.* 1986 **6**: 139–219.
26. Craig A. D. Heppleman B. & Schaible H. -G, The projection of the medial and posterior articular nerves of the cat's knee to the spinal cord. *J. Comp. Neurol.* 1988 **276**: 279–88.
27. Cervero F. & Tattersall E. H. Somatic and visceral sensory integration in the thoracic spinal cord. *Progr. Brain Res.* 1986; **67**: 189–205.
28. Sugiura Y., Terui N., Hosoya Y. & Kohno K. Distribution of unmyelinated primary afferent fibres in the dorsal horn. In: *Processing of Sensory Information in the Superficial Dorsal Horn of the Spinal Cord.* Cervero F., Bennett G. J. & Headley P. M. (eds) New York: Plenum Press, 1989 15–27.
29. Cervero F. & Connell L. A. Fine afferent from viscera do not terminate in the substantia gelantinosa of the thoracic spinal cord. *Brain Res.* 1984; **294**: 370–74.
30. Ruda M. A., Bennett G. J., & Dubner R. Neurochemistry and neural circuitry in the dorsal dorn. *Progr. Brain Res.* 1986 **66**: 219–68.
31. Jessell T. M. & Iversen L. L. Opiate analgesics inhibit substance P release from rat trigeminal nucleus. *Nature* 1977 **268**: 549–51.
32. Sharkey K. A., Sobrino J. A., & Cervero F. Visceral and somatic origin of calcitonin-gene-related-peptide-immunoreactivity in the superficial and deep laminae of the thoracic spinal cord of the rat. In: *Processing of Sensory Information in the Superficial Dorsal Horn of the Spinal Cord.* Cervero F., Bennett J. & Headley P. M. (eds) New York: Plenum Press, 1989 99–102.
33. Ruda M.A., Cohen L., Shiosoria S., Takahashio, Allen B., Humphrey E.m and Iadorola M. J., *In situ* hybridisation, histochemical and immunocytochemical analysis of opioid gene products in a rat model of peripheral inflammation. In *Processing of Sensory Information in the*

Superficial Dorsal Horn of the Spinal Cord. Cervero, F., Bennet, G. J. and Headley, P.M. (eds. New York, Plenum Press, 1989, 383–94).

34. Besson J. -M., Lombard M. C., Zamac J. M., Besse D., Peschanski M. & Roques B. P. Opioid receptors in the dorsal horn of intact and deafferented rats: autoradiographic and electrophysiological studies. In: *Processing of Sensory Information in the Superficial Dorsal Horn of the Spinal Cord.* Cervero F., Bennett G. J. & Headley P. M. (eds. New York: Plenum Press, 1989; 415–28.

35. Bennett G. J., Kajander K. C., Sahara Y., Iadarola M. A. & Sugimoto T. Neurochemical and anatomical changes in the dorsal horn of rats with an experimental painful peripheral neuropathy. In: *Processing of Sensory Information in the Superficial Dorsal Horn of the Spinal Cord.* Cervero F., Bennett G. J., Headley P. M. (eds) New York: Plenum Press 1989: 463–72

36. LeBars D. & Chitour D. Do convergent neurones in the dorsal horn discriminate nociceptive from non-nociceptive information? *Pain* 1983 **17**: 1–19.

37. Mendell L. M. Physiological properties of unmyelinated fibre projections to the spinal cord *Exp. Neurol.* 1966 **16**: 316–32.

38. Laird, J. M. A. & Cervero F., A comparative study of the changes in receptive field properties of multireceptive and nocireceptive rat dorsal horn neurones following noxious mechanical stimulation. *J. Neurophysiol.* 1989 **62**: 854–63.

39. McMahon S. B. & Wall P. D. (1984). The receptive fields of rat lamina I projection cells move to incorporate a nearby region of injury. *Pain,* 1984; **19**: 235–47.

40. Hylden J. L. K. Nahin R. L., Traub R. J. & Dubner, R. Expansion of receptive fields of spinal lamina 1 projection neurones in rats with unilateral adjuvant-induced inflammation: the contribution of central dorsal horn mechanisms. *Pain* 1989 **37**: 229–43.

41. Schaible H. -G., Schmidt R. F. & Willis W. D. Enhancement of the responses of ascending tract cells in the cat spinal cord by acute inflammation of the knee joint. *Exp. Brain Res.,* 1987 **66**: 489–99

42. Woolf C. J. & King A. E. Subliminal fringes and the plasticity of dorsal horn neurones receptive field properties. *Soc. for Neurosci. Abstr.* 1988 **14**: 696

43. Simone D. A., Baumann T. K., Collins J. G. & Lamotte R. H. Sensitization of cat dorsal horn neurons to innocuous mechanical stimulation after intradermal injection of capsaicin. *Brain Res.* 1989 **486**: 185–89.

44. Hoheisel U. & Mense S. Long-term changes in discharge behaviour of cat dorsal horn neurones following noxious stimulation of deep tissues. *Pain* 1989 **36**: 239–47.

45. Cook, A. J. Woolf C. J. Wall P. D. & McMahon S. B. Dynamic receptive field plasticity in rat spinal cord dorsal horn following C-primary afferent input. *Nature,* 1987 **325**: 151–3.

46. Menetrey, D. & Besson, J. -M. Electrophysiological characteristics of dorsal horn cells in rats with cutaneous inflammation resulting from chronic arthritis. *Pain* 1982 **13**: 343–64.

47. Snow, P. J. & Wilson, P. Denervation induced changes in somatotopic organisation: the ineffective projections of afferent fibres and structural plasticity. In *Processing of Sensory Information in the Superficial Dorsal Horn*

of the Spinal Cord. Cervero, F., Bennett, G. J. & Headley, P. M. (eds) New York: Plenum Press, 1989 285–306.

48. LeBars D., Calvino B., Villanueva L. & Cadden S. Physiological approaches to counter-irritation phenomena. In: *Stress-induced Analgesia*. Tricklebank M. D. & Curzon G. (eds) Chichester, Wiley: 1984 67–101.

49. Basbaum A. I. & Fields H. L. Endogenous pain control mechanisms: review and hypothesis. *Ann. Neurol.* 1978; **4**: 451–62.

50. Basbaum A. I. & Fields H. L. Endogenous pain control systems: brainstem spinal pathways and endorphin circuitry. *Ann. Rev. Neurosci.* 1984; **7**: 309–38.

51. Willis W. D. Control of nociceptive transmission in the spinal cord. *Progr. Sens Physiol.* 1982 **3**: 1–155.

52. Duggan A. W. Pharmacology of descending control systems. *Phil. Trans.*, R. Soc. Lond. B. 1985 **308**: 375–91.

53. Clarke R. W. & Matthews B. The effects of analgesics and remote noxious stimuli on the jaw-opening reflex evoked by tooth-pulp stimulation in the cat. *Brain Res.* 1985 **327**: 105–11.

54. Cervero F. & Wolstencroft J. H. A positive feedback loop between spinal cord nociceptive pathways and antinociceptive areas of the cat's brain stem *Pain* 1984, **20**: 125–38.

2

Mechanism of impulse block

B. G. Covino

Pain may be modified or inhibited by (1) modulating the perception of pain impulses arriving in the brain, (2) altering the release or action of nociceptive neurotransmitters in the spinal cord, or (3) inhibiting the conduction of painful impulses in peripheral sensory nerves prior to entering the dorsal horn within the spinal cord. Blockade of sensory impulses in peripheral nerves can be achieved by various physical, chemical or mechanical methods. However, clinically, impulse blockade in peripheral nerves is usually achieved by the use of local anaesthetic agents. This chapter will concern itself with a review of the current theories concerning the mechanism of conduction blockade produced by local anaesthetic agents.

Anatomy of peripheral nerve

Peripheral nerves are mixed nerves containing both myelinated and unmyelinated fibres which conduct afferent and efferent impulses subserving either sensory or motor functions, (Fig. 2.1). The entire nerve is surrounded by an epineurium, or sheath, composed of connective tissue and tightly joined cells. Within this sheath, groups of nerve fibres are organized in fascicles surrounded by a second sheath, the perineurium. Finally, each individual axon is intimately surrounded by non-nuronal glial cells which form the endoneurium.

These various neuronal coverings serve as barriers which can influence the diffusion of local anaesthetics. The A and B nerve fibres are encased in a myelin sheath which extends, discontinuously, from the roots of the spinal cord to the region of entry at the target organ. Each segment or internode of myelin is formed by one Schwann cell that wraps around the axon, forming an insulating cylinder of as many as several hundred bilayer membranes. The myelin sheath of peripheral fibres accounts for more than half the thickness of the fibre diameter. The myelin sheath is interrupted at intervals by narrow zones of constrictions, i.e. the nodes of Ranvier, that contain the structural elements essential for neuronal excitability (Fig. 2.1). These nodes are covered by a Schwann cell that projects to the surface of the axolemma and makes several intimate contacts with the neuronal surface. The sodium channels of myelinated fibres are located at the nodes of Ranvier such that excitation proceeds from one node to the next. The potassium channels are present almost exclusively in the internodal region where they exert little influence on impulse propagation. Between the extra-nodal Schwann cell and the axolemma lies nodal-gap substance, dense in negatively charged material, which may act as a reservoir to bind metal cations and basic drugs near the nodal membrane. Thus, at no point along the fibre is the axon membrane freely exposed to the surrounding medium.

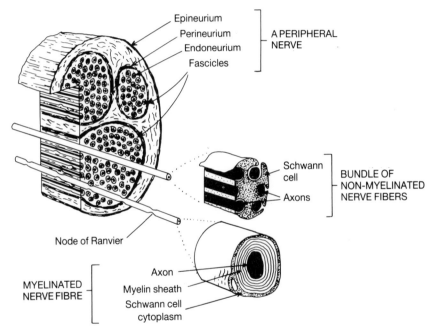

Figure 2.1   Anatomy of peripheral nerve.

All fibres of diameter greater than 1 micron are myelinated. Small C fibers are unmyelinated but are enclosed within a Schwann cell that forms an intimate cover around several fibres. Cross-sectional electron micrographs of non-myelinated nerves show that individual axons are located adjacent to the periphery of such a bundle circumscribing the large nucleus of the Schwann cell. The Schwann cell's plasmalemma encloses each axon separately, folding the cytoplasm of the supporting cell around most of the axon's diameter. Any one axon passes sequentially from one encasing Schwann cell to another with no apparent interruptions. The structural association between neuron and glia is maintained along the entire length of the fibre and may be functionally similar to that of the myelinated axon and its enclosing Schwann cell at each node of Ranvier.

The plasma membrane of nerve cells consists of densely staining outer surfaces, spaced 7.5–10nm apart, which enclose a relatively electron-transparent medium. Myelinated and unmyelinated nerve fibres have the same general morphology although the membrane has characteristic features in specialized regions, such as at sensory nerve endings, and at the synapses.

Morphological and electrical studies demonstrate that nerve membranes are mainly lipid bilayers encasing proteins, some of which permit ions to pass through a hydrocarbon interior of otherwise high resistance (Fig. 2.2). Both proteins and lipids in membranes are often associated with complex carbohydrate structures, located on the extracellular side of the membrane, and the proteins may also interact with the carbohydrates of the internal cytoskeleton. The emerging picture is one of a biosynthetically dynamic structure, where membrane proteins not only move about within the membrane, but are being continuously synthesized, inserted and removed throughout the life of the neuron.

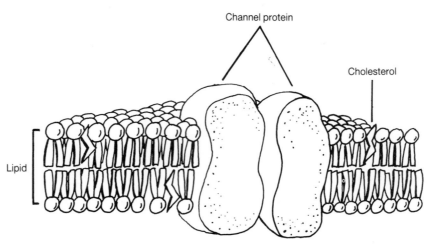

Figure 2.2   Structure of nerve membrane.

The lipid composition of the nerve membrane influences its structural and dynamic characteristics, and modulates the activities of some of the intrinsically bound enzymes. It also regulates the rate and potency of action of various drugs. The morphological and electrical properties of nerve membranes are quite similar to those of lipid bilayers which contain some protein or other ion-transporting substance. Direct structural determinations of nerve membranes by X-ray diffraction further support the bilayer model. Studies of bilayers made from lipid extracted from nerves provide data comparable with those characteristic of pure lipid bilayers.

Membranes are composed of phospholipids, cholesterol, proteins and carbohydrates, which are usually conjugated with other substances to form glycoproteins or glycolipids. Protein accounts for more than 30 per cent of non-myelinated nerve dry weight, yet most of it is localized at the membrane surface and not within the hydrocarbon region. Cholesterol is interdigitated among the phospholipids and influences their behaviour. When X-ray patterns of bilayers made only from phospholipids are compared with those made from total lipid extract, the inclusion of cholesterol appears to increase the separation of polar lipid headgroups in the bilayer to that seen in the axolemma and causes an increase in the parallel orientation of the fatty acid chains of phospholipids. The presence of cholesterol increases the degree of order in the membrane.

Despite their orderly alignment in the plane of the membrane, neural lipids behave like fluid components within the membrane. The fluidity in nerve membranes can be detected by electron spin resonance (ESR). 'Spin labels' are dissolved in the hydrocarbon phase, or covalently bound to molecules which become oriented in the membrane. Spin-label studies show that the hydrocarbon region of nerve membranes is very fluid at physiological temperatures. The fatty acid tails of membrane lipids are rotating and bending at frequencies up to 10^9 s^{-1}. ESR signals from long-chain acids spin-labelled at different positions along the hydrocarbon chain indicate that the nerve membranes in which they are inserted are mostly fluid and have the least degree of orientation near the centre of the hydrocarbon region. The fluidity decreases while the degree of orientation increases as the label is moved closer to the polar headgroup region of the lipids. Thus, there is far more motion in the centre of a membrane than near the aqueous interface. This is of particular interest because local anaesthetics appear to distribute in lipid bilayer membranes between the fatty acid core and the phospholipid headgroup region adjacent to extracellular and cytoplasmic solutions.

Electrophysiology of peripheral nerve

At rest a negative electrical potential of approximately –60 to –90 mV exists across the nerve cell membrane which represents the resting membrane potential. If a stimulus of sufficient intensity is applied to the nerve, the interior of the cell becomes progressively less negative with respect to the exterior, resulting in a state of depolarization (Fig. 2.3). The cell membrane possesses a critical threshold potential or firing level which must be achieved before complete depolarization can occur. Normally, the threshold potential level is approximately 20 mV less than the resting

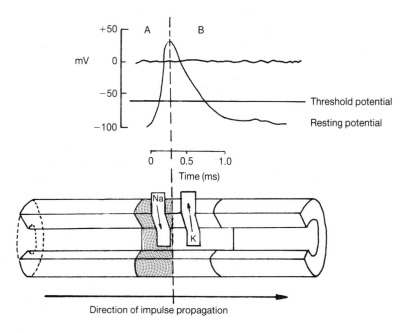

Figure 2.3   Action potential from peripheral nerve (upper) and ion fluxes association with action potential (lower). A represents depolarization phase and B represents repolarization phase.

potential. If the stimulus applied to the nerve is not sufficient to decrease the potential difference across the cell membrane from the resting level to the threshold level, then a localized incomplete state of depolarization occurs which is not adequate to produce a propagated action potential. Once the threshold potential level is achieved, an extremely rapid phase of depolarization commences, which is spontaneous in nature and not dependent on the strength of the applied stimulus. The nerve membrane essentially follows the 'all or none' rule, i.e. an applied stimulus of sufficient strength is required to achieve the threshold potential level which, in turn, will result in complete depolarization (Fig. 2.3). Any additional increase in stimulus intensity has no effect on the degree of depolarization or the amplitude of the action potential. Complete depolarization of the cell membrane results in a reversal of the electrical potential, such that at the end of the depolarization phase, the interior of the cell actually has a positive electrical potential of +40 mV as compared to the exterior of the cell. Under normal conditions the height of the action potential is approximately 110 mV, i.e. the potential difference across the membrane has changed from a resting potential level of –70 mV to a peak level of +40 mV at the end of depolarization.

At the conclusion of the depolarization phase, repolarization of the cell membrane begins. During this time period, the electrical potential within the cell again becomes progressively more negative until such time as the original resting potential of –60 to –90 mV is re-established. The period of repolarization is important eletrophysiologically since during this phase the membrane is in a state of refractoriness. During the early portion of the repolarization phase, the refractoriness is absolute in nature such that the cell will not respond to a stimulus regardless of strength. During the latter phase of repolarization the cell is in a state of relative refractoriness. During this time period the cell will only respond to a stimulus whose intensity is greater than that normally required to produce depolarization. The refractory period is important, since it limits the number of impulses that can be conducted along a nerve fibre per unit time. The entire process of depolarization and repolarization occurs within 1 ms. The depolarization phase occupies approximately 30 per cent of the entire action potential, whereas repolarization accounts for the remaining 70 per cent. Frequently a brief period of hyperpolarization may be observed following the end of the repolarization phase. During this time, the potential difference across the cell membrane is actually more negative than during the resting potential.

Propagation of the action potential from the area of initial excitation along the entire length of a nerve fibre does not require sequential stimulation of individual segments of the nerve. Once initial excitation occurs in a localized area of the nerve, a spontaneous and self-perpetuating system propagates the impulse along the entire length of the nerve fibre. This process is dependent on the change of electrical potential across the cell membrane at the area of excitation and the ability of the nerve to function as an electrical cable. In unmyelinated C fibres, current will flow from the depolarized action region into the adjacent polarized segment (Fig. 2.4). This current flow will thereby reduce the charge and voltage in the inactive region, which is sufficient to decrease the intracellular potential to the threshold level required for depolarization. Therefore, the local circuit flow of current between immediate adjacent areas of polarized and depolarized membrane results in spontaneous propagation of the impulse along the fibre at a constant velocity of approximately 1 m.s^{-1}. In myelinated nerve fibers, the local circuit current spreads along the length of the nerve activating many nodes of Ranvier. The conduction velocity is proportional to the size of the fibre and intranodal distances. Thus, in large myelinated A fibres impulse propagation occurs at the rate of 70–120 m.s^{-1} while small lightly myelinated B fibres conduct impulses at the rate of 3–15 m.s^{-1}.

Ionic factors responsible for action potential

The electrophysiological properties of the nerve membrane are dependent on (a) the concentration of electrolytes in nerve cytoplasm and extracellular

Impulse direction

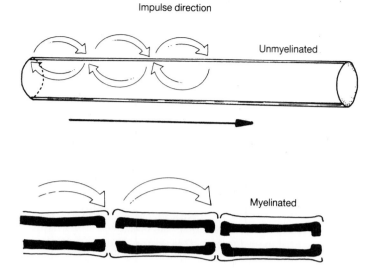

Figure 2.4   Current flow and impulse propagation in unmyelinated (upper) and myelinated (lower) fibres.

fluid, and (b) the permeability of the cell membrane to various ions, particularly sodium and potassium. The ionic composition of the cytoplasm and the extracellular fluid differ markedly. The intracellular concentration of potassium is approximately 110 to 170 M.l^{-1}, whereas the intracellular concentration of sodium and chloride ions is approximately 5–10 M.l^{-1}. In extracellular fluid the situation is reversed. The concentration of sodium is approximately 140 M.l^{-1} and the concentration of chloride is 110 M.l^{-1}. On the other hand, the extracellular concentration of potassium is only 3–5 M.l^{-1}. The ionic asymmetry on either side of the cell membrane is due in part to the selective permeability characteristics of the membrane. At rest, potassium ions may diffuse easily across the cell membrane indicating that the membrane is fully permeable to this particular ion. However, only limited diffusion of sodium ions across the membrane occurs at rest indicating that the membrane is relatively impermeable to sodium, which accounts for the high extracellular concentration and low intracellular concentration of sodium. Although the membrane is permeable to potassium ions, a high intracellular concentration of this ion is maintained by the attractive forces of the negative charges, mainly on proteins which exist within the cell. These large negatively-charged proteins are unable to diffuse across the cell membrane. The attraction of the negative charges on the proteins tends to counter-balance the tendency of the positively-charged potassium ions to diffuse out of the cell by passive movement along a concentration gradient and through a freely permeable membrane. The electrical potential which exists across a membrane separating two concentrations of the same ion is predicted by the Nernst equation.

$$E = \frac{RT \ln [A]_i}{nF [A]_o}$$

Where E = membrane potential between inside and outside of cell

R = gas constant in joules (8.315)

T = absolute temperature

n = valence of the ion

F = Faraday's constant (96,500 coulombs)

ln = natural logarithm

at room temperature $18\frac{1}{2}°C$ and assuming a K_i/K_o ratio across the nerve membrane of 30, the Nernst equation would predict the following.

$$E = -58 \log \frac{[30K]_i}{[K]_o}$$

$$E = -85.7 \text{ mV}$$

This predicted resting membrane potential of –85.7 mV agrees closely with the measured resting potential values of –60 to –90 mV obtained from nerve preparations with intracellular electrodes. At rest, it would appear that the nerve cell behaves as a potassium electrode, which should react to changes in intra- or extracellular potassium concentration. It has been shown that changes in the intracellular or extracellular concentration of potassium will markedly alter the resting membrane potential. For example, as the extracellular concentration of potassium is increased, the resting membrane potential will tend to decrease. Studies have indicated that a decrease of 58 mV in resting potential occurs for a 10-fold change in external potassium concentration. On the other hand, changes in sodium concentration appear to have little, if any, effect on the resting membrane potential.

Excitation of a nerve results in marked changes in the permeability of the cell membrane and ionic fluxes across the membrane. The movement of ions across the nerve membrane occurs through ion-specific pores or channels. Sodium channels have been studied most extensively. Efforts have been made to determine the size and density of these channels. In addition, physiologic studies have indicated that sodium channels exist in various states.[2] When the nerve membrane is quiescent the sodium channels are considered to be in a state of rest (R), and impermeable to the passage of sodium ions (Fig. 2.5). Following stimulation, the channels pass from a closed to an open state (O), thus permitting the passage of sodium ions across the membrane. When the threshold potential is exceeded most of the sodium channels are in an open state allowing a

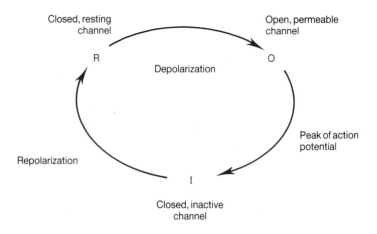

Figure 2.5   Various states of sodium channel prior to and following membrane activation.

maximum increase in the permeability of the cell membrane to sodium ions and an explosively rapid influx of sodium ions into the axoplasm follows. This marked increase of sodium conductance is responsible for the rapid depolarization of the cell. As the potential difference changes from the threshold level of approximately –50 mV to +40 mV at the peak of the action potential, the open sodium channels become inactivated (I) leading to a decrease in sodium permeability. It is this sodium inactivation that ultimately terminates the depolarization phase. At the end of depolarization or at the peak of the action potential, the nerve membrane is essentially transformed from a potassium electrode to a sodium electrode, and the positive membrane potential of +40 mV can be calculated again from the Nernst equation by substituting the ratio of sodium ions between the inside and the outside of the nerve membrane (Na_i/Na_o) for the potassium ion ratio (K_i/K_o).

At the conclusion of the depolarization phase, the membrane starts to repolarize. The initial phase of repolarization and the absolute refractory period is related mainly to inactivation of sodium channels (I) resulting in a decrease in sodium flux. However, the remaining portion of the repolarization phase is a function of an increase in potassium conductance and efflux of this ion from the interior to the exterior of the cell. Potassium conductance is still somewhat greater than normal when repolarization is complete, which accounts for the phase of membrane hyperpolarization. When the membrane potential returns to its normal resting level, then potassium and sodium channels have also returned to their normal resting states.

Although the fluxes of sodium and potassium are high during the depolarization and repolarization phases, the actual concentration changes across the cell membrane are very small, because the time during which these flows occur is very short. Therefore, following return of the membrane to the resting potential level, only a slight excess of sodium ions is present within the cell and a slight excess of potassium ions exists outside of the nerve cell. At the conclusion of the excitation period, a metabolically active period begins, although electrically the nerve cell is quiescent. Restoration of the normal ionic gradient across the nerve membrane requires the expenditure of energy for the active transport of sodium from the inside to the outside of the nerve cell against a concentration gradient. This active transport of sodium ions is made possible by so-called 'sodium pump'. The energy required to drive the sodium pump is derived from the oxidative metabolism of adenosine triphosphate. This metabolic pump, which actively extrudes intracellular sodium ions, is also believed responsible, in part, for the transport of potassium ions from the extracellular space to the interior of the nerve cell.

The return of potassium to the interior of the nerve cell occurs against a concentration gradient, but down an electrogenic gradient. Thus, re-establishment of the potassium gradient across the cell membrane may be partly an active process and partly a passive phenomenon. Potassium will continue to return to the interior of the cell until the electrostatic attraction of the negative charges on the intracellular proteins balances the chemical concentration gradient. Figure 2.3 summarizes the relationship between electrical activity in the nerve and the alterations in ionic fluxes across the membrane.

Mechanism of local anaesthetic induced conduction blockade

Application of a sufficient concentration of local anaesthetic agent to peripheral nerve either *in vitro* or *in vivo* will inhibit impulse conduction. However, electrophysiological studies have shown that neither the resting membrane potential nor the threshold potential of isolated nerves is altered following exposure to various concentrations of local anaesthetic agents, such as procaine or lignocaine.

The primary effect of local anaesthetic agents involves the depolarization phase of the action potential. A decrease in the rate and degree of depolarization is observed as the concentration of local anaesthetic agent applied to an isolated nerve is increased. Although a subminimal concentration of local anaesthetic agents will not prevent the development of a propagated action potential, rate of depolarization and repolarization is decreased, refractory period is prolonged and conduction velocity is decreased. As a result, the number of impulses transmitted per unit time in an isolated nerve exposed to a subminimal concentration of local anaesthetic agent will be decreased. When the minimum concentration (Cm) of a local anaesthetic agent required to cause complete conduction blockade is achieved, then the rate and degree of depolarization is sufficiently depressed that the threshold potential level is not achieved. Studies by Aceves and Machne[3] have shown a 59 per cent decrease in the maximum rate of rise of the action potential of the isolated lumbar spinal ganglion of the frog after exposure to procaine. Similarly, Shanes *et al.*[4] reported a 42 per cent decrease in the maximum rate of depolarization of the squid axon following the application of cocaine or procaine. In both studies, a concomitant decrease in the rate of repolarization of 37–55 per cent was also observed. The prolonged repolarization phase may reflect a direct local anaesthetic action or may be indicative of a direct relationship between the rate of repolarization and the rate of depolarization. In general the primary action of local anaesthetic is a decrease in the rate and degree of depolarization.

Since the action potential of the nerve membrane is a function of changes in sodium and potassium permeability and conductance, a number of studies have been carried out to evaluate the effect of local anaesthetics on ionic permeability. Initially, Condouris[5] observed a direct correlation between the concentration of sodium in the bathing solution and the concentration of cocaine required to reduce the height of the spike potential of the isolated frog sciatic–peroneal nerve trunk. For example, at a normal sodium concentration of 116 mmol, approximately 3.2 mmoles of cocaine were required to produce a 50 per cent decrease in the height of the spike potential. When the sodium concentration was lowered to 12 mmoles, only 0.15 mmol of cocaine were necessary to cause a similar reduction of 50 per cent in the amplitude of the spike potential.

The most direct evidence concerning the effect of local anaesthetic agents on sodium and potassium conductance has been obtained by means of voltage clamp techniques. Taylor[6] and Shanes et al.[4] demonstrated that procaine and cocaine are capable of decreasing the inward flow of sodium currents and the outward flow of potassium currents during voltage clamping of the membrane. However, both studies demonstrated a greater inhibitory effect on sodium conductance (g_{Na}) than on potassium conductance (g_K). For example, 0.05–0.1 per cent cocaine produced a 31–64 per cent decrease in g_{Na} compared to a 22–57 per cent decrease in g_K. Procaine (0.1 per cent) resulted in a 58 per cent decrease in g_{Na} while at the same time reducing g_K by 21 per cent. Furthermore, studies on the isolated frog sciatic nerve by Hille[7] in which the membrane potential was held at the normal resting potential of –75 mV demonstrated complete loss of sodium currents in the presence of $10^{-3}M$ lignocaine with no discernible effect on outward potassium current. A concentration of 3.5×10^{-3} M of lignocaine was required to produce a 25 per cent decrease in g_K. In a subsequent study, Strichartz[8] also demonstrated almost complete inhibition of g_{Na} with minimal change in g_K following application of lignocaine to a single myelinated frog sciatic nerve preparation.

Definitive proof that local anaesthetic induced conduction blockade is due to an inhibition of sodium conductance was forthcoming from investigations with the biotoxins, tetrodotoxin and saxitoxin. These two substances are the most potent nerve conduction blockers found to date. Tetrodotoxin will prevent excitation of the isolated squid axon at a concentration of 10^{-7} M. In terms of ionic membrane permeability, these two biotoxins have been demonstrated in various biological preparations to specifically inhibit sodium conductance without any effect on potassium conductance. For example, Hille[7,9] reported that $3{\times}10^{-7}$ M tetrodotoxin completely inhibited g_{Na} in the isolated frog sciatic nerve without any discernible effect on g_K. Similarly, saxitoxin caused a dose-related decrease in g_{Na} with complete blockade occurring at approximately 10^{-7} M, while no change in g_K was observed at any concentration of saxitoxin.

In summary, the basic mechanism by which local anaesthetics cause conduction block in peripheral nerves involves inhibition of the increase in membrane permeability to sodium ions which results in a failure of membrane depolarization.

Site of action of local anaesthetic agents

In recent years attempts have been made to determine the specific site in the nerve membrane at which local anaesthetics exert their inhibitory action. Three specific sites have been suggested as possible locations for the action of local anaesthetics

(1)   the surface of the nerve membrane;
(2)   within the nerve membrane; and
(3)   specific receptors within the sodium channel.

Membrane surface location

About 15 per cent of the neuronal phospholipids carry net negative charges: the charged species are phosphatidylserine and phosphatidylinositol. These lipids may alter membrane excitability and also modulate the uptake of basic amine local anaesthetics. Many studies have shown that fixed charges near sodium channels in nerve can influence excitability. Such fixed charges create electric potentials at the membrane surface which contribute to the electric field in the membrane, and thus influence the 'voltage sensors' which control ion permeability channels. A membrane with negative charges fixed to its surface tends to accumulate cations and repel anions in the adjacent solution. In turn, the presence of cations, particularly multivalent cations, e.g. Ca^{2+}, decreases the local surface potential due to ion accumulation and in this way can influence excitability. For example, increasing external Ca^{2+} raises the firing threshold of nerves, and this is explained by a change of the surface electric potential that in turn changes the electric field within the membrane which is detected by 'voltage sensors' of ion channels as being equivalent to a hyperpolarization of the nerve. The Ca^{2+} ions need not interact directly with the ion channels, according to this mechanism.

Negative charges fixed at membrane surfaces also attract protonated local anaesthetics and thus increase their adsorption to the membrane and so decrease the negativity of the surface of the nerve membrane. The electrostatic interactions between membrane negative charges, local anaesthetics, and Ca^{2+} ions account for the binding competition observed in experimental studies. However, certain pharmacological actions cannot be explained by such electrostatic competition. For example, elevated extracellular Ca^{2+} antagonizes the inhibition from uncharged benzocaine. In addition, quaternary forms of local anaesthetics can absorb to the outer surface of bilayer membranes changing the potential by 10 mV, yet have no effect on nerve excitability when restricted to the extracellular solution.[10] Therefore, local anaesthetics must exert specific effects other than those due to electrostatic interactions, but these interactions can modulate the biological effects of the anaesthetics.

Location within the nerve membrane

The highly lipid nature of the nerve membrane and the relationship between local anaesthetic potency and lipid solubility has led some investigators to conclude that the site of action of local anaesthetic agents resides within the lipid component of the nerve membrane. Seeman[11] studied a number of different agents capable of producing conduction blockade and reported an inverse correlation between the membrane/buffer partition coefficient of the agents and the concentration required in the membrane to cause conduction block.

An intramembranal site of action of local anaesthetic agents is visualized as causing some type of confirmational change in the organization of the membrane. The alteration most commonly postulated is membrane expansion or change in critical volume. The membrane expansion theory of local anaesthesia is basically an extension of the Meyer-Overton law for general anaesthesia, which stated that the physico-chemical combination of an anaesthetic substance with cell lipids causes a change in the relationship between cell constituents which, in turn, leads to an inhibition of cell function. Originally the membrane expansion theory of local anaesthesia suggested a constriction of the sodium channels due to increased lateral pressure within the membrane. *In vitro* studies by Skou[12] in which the surface pressure of monomolecular layers of lipids increased following placement of local anaesthetics into the solution below the lipid layer served as the basis for this concept of lateral expansion within the membrane. Seeman[11] has attempted to quantify the actual change in volume of membranes during conditions of local anaesthesia. In general, membrane concentrations of 0.04 mol. kg^{-1} of membrane are required for the production of conduction blockade. This concentration occupies a volume of 0.3 per cent of the membrane which results in a 2–3 per cent expansion of the membrane. The membrane expansion theory would readily explain the site and mechanism of action of local anaesthetic agents that exist only in an uncharged form such as benzocaine and benzyl alcohol. Moreover, it would also provide a single theory for the site and mechanism of action of both general and local anaesthetic drugs. With regard to general anaesthetic agents, one of the critical experiments that has been quoted to support the concept of membrane expansion or increase in volume involves reversal of anaesthesia by exposure to elevated atmospheric pressures. This can be dramatically demonstrated in the following fashion: the addition of general anaesthetics to a bath containing tadpoles abolishes the spontaneous swimming of the tadpoles. When the bath containing the anaesthetized tadpoles is exposed to hydrostatic pressures of 150 to 350 atmospheres, swimming motion is again re-established indicating a removal of the state of anaesthesia. In addition, emulsions of general anaesthetics can produce conduction block in a variety of peripheral nerves, which can then be antagonized by an increase in atmospheric pressure. Similar studies with local anaesthetic agents are limited and contradictory in nature. Roth, Smith and Paton[13] reported that high pressure could reverse the depression of action potential amplitude in frog sciatic nerves produced by chloroform, diethyl ether and halothane. However, no pressure-induced antagonism of action potential depression due to procaine or dibucaine was observed. Similar studies were conducted by Kendig and Cohen[14] utilizing the preganglionic sympathetic nerve of the superior cervical ganglion of the rat. Depression of action potential amplitude was induced following exposure to the general anaesthetics, halothane and methoxyflurane, the local anaesthetics, lignocaine, procaine and benzocaine, the biotoxin, tetrodotoxin, a quaternary amine analog of lignocaine, QX-572, and the spin-label molecule, TEMPO. Subsequent exposure of the blocked nerves to high pressure helium resulted in partial, but significant antagonism of the halothane, methoxyflurane, benzocaine, lignocaine and TEMPO induced action potential depression. However, no pressure reversal of procaine, QX-572 or tetrodotoxin induced depression was observed.

These findings are consistent with the hypothesis that conduction blockade may be related, in part, to membrane expansion following penetration of the uncharged form of local anaesthetic into the interior of the cell membrane. Since QX-572 and tetrodotoxin exist only in a charged form, these agents presumably are incapable of membrane expansion. The absence of pressure antagonism to procaine is probably related to the high pK$_a$ of this agent, which means that at a pH of 7.4, less than 5 per cent of procaine exists in an uncharged form. These findings[14] differ from the results of Boggs *et al.*[15] who utilized the rat phrenic nerve and desheathed frog sciatic nerve to study the interaction of high pressure and local anaesthetic blockade. The spin-label molecule, TEMPO, produced a 68 per cent decrease in action potential amplitude at normal atmospheric pressure. Upon application of helium at a pressure of 100 atmospheres, a further reduction of 14 per cent in action potential height occurred. High pressure had no observable effect on the action potential depression produced by lignocaine and benyzl alcohol. Thus, it appears that high pressure may enhance, antagonize, or exert no effect on conduction blockade produced in peripheral nerves by various local anaesthetic substances.

A number of modifications of the membrane expansion theory have been proposed all of which are based on an intramembrane site of anaesthetic action. A variety of experimental techniques, including nuclear magnetic resonance, have been employed to study changes in the fluidity of model membranes following exposure to local anaesthetic agents. Phospholipid membranes may undergo a transition from a gel crystalline to a liquid crystalline state. Various clinically useful local anaesthetics such as procaine, lignocaine, amethocaine and bupivacaine have been shown to increase the fluidity of these phospholipid membranes. This increase in the freedom of movement of lipid molecules within the membrane may occur with or without a concomitant increase in the volume of the membrane. For example, the increase in fluidity or disorder of the lipid molecules may result in conformational changes in the membrane proteins which are closely associated with the lipids. The concept of increased fluidity of lipid molecules resulting either in an expansion of the membrane or a confirmational change in membrane proteins is consistent with the fluid mosaic membrane model proposed by Singer.[16]

Irrespective of the precise membrane perturbation produced by local anaesthetics, the common feature of these various theories involves a decrease in the diameter of the sodium channel, or a prevention of sodium channel opening upon membrane activation. Therefore, the local anaesthetics are perceived as penetrating the interior of the cell membrane, producing a confirmational change in the membrane which maintains the sodium channels in a closed state resulting in a decreased sodium permeability and, ultimately, conduction blockade. Although the site of local anaesthetic action within the nerve membrane is attractive from a theoretical point of view, it is difficult to prove experimentally that membrane confirmational changes can produce conduction blockade. In addition, although the suggestive evidence is strong that uncharged forms of local anaesthetics may act from within the cell membrane, the data are not equally strong regarding charged local anaesthetics. Finally, some data exist with indicate that local anaesthetics stabilize and inhibit confirmational changes in certain membranes (rat liver mitochondria) rather than inducing alterations in membrane configuration.

Specific receptor sites within the sodium channel

The third and most common site proposed for the action of local anaesthetic agents involves specific receptors within the sodium channel. The concept of a specific receptor site for local anaesthetic activity is based on the following information: (1) *in vitro* biochemical evidence that local anaesthetic agents can bind to phospholipids and/or proteins; (2) specificity of optical isomers of local anaesthetic drugs; (3) selectivity of binding of the biotoxins, tetrodotoxin and saxitoxin; and (4) modulation of local anaesthesia by the frequency of nerve stimulation.

In vitro binding studies
It has been demonstrated that local anaesthetic agents are capable of binding both to phospholipids and proteins. Feinstein[17] has suggested that one local anaesthetic molecule may serve as an electrostatic bond between the negatively charged phosphate groups of two phospholipid molecules. In addition, evidence exists for the formation of hydrogen bonds between local anaesthetics and phospholipids. Protein binding of local anaesthetics has also been well documented. Studies on nerve homogenates revealed that approximately 75 per cent of amethocaine is bound to proteins as compared to 6 per cent for procaine. Subsequent studies with plasma proteins have shown that all amide-type local anaesthetics are capable of binding to protein, but to varying degrees. A direct correlation exists between the degree of protein binding and the duration of conduction blockade. For example, action potentials recorded from the surface of an isolated frog sciatic nerve are depressed by 50 per cent following exposure to 20 mM of lignocaine but return to their control height within 30 minutes following removal of lignocaine from the bathing solution. Similar experiments with bupivacaine or etidocaine show that approximately two hours is required for complete reversal of conduction blockade. In terms of protein binding, lignocaine is 55 per cent bound to plasma protein, while bupivacaine and etidocaine are 95 per cent protein bound. These studies do not prove that local anaesthetics combine with a specific receptor in the membrane. Nevertheless, the fact that these agents can bind to lipoproteins, the lipoprotein composition of the nerve membrane and the relationship between protein binding and anaesthetic activity are certainly suggestive of a local anaesthetic–lipoprotein receptor interaction.

Specificity of optical isomers of local anaesthetics
Akerman[18] studied the optical isomers of a series of different local anaesthetics including certain agents which are employed clinically, e.g. prilocaine, mepivacaine, and bupivacaine. It was shown, for example, that the levo form of prilocaine was twice as potent as the dextro form in terms of producing corneal anaesthesia in rabbits and cutaneous anaesthesia in guinea pigs. Studies on the isolated sheathed and desheathed frog sciatic

nerve showed as much as a 5-fold difference in conduction blocking activity between the isomers of different local anaesthetics, e.g. levo-bupivacaine was approximately four times more potent than dextro-bupivacaine. The most detailed study concerning site and mechanism of action of optical isomers was carried out with an experimental compound, RAC 109. This local anaesthetic substance is a succinimide derivative in contrast to an agent such as lignocaine which is an anilide derivative. The enantiomers of RAC 109 were designated simply RAC 109 I and RAC 109 II. Although the absolute configuration of these two isomers is not known, they do possess opposite steric configurations. Measurements of the maximum rate of rise of the action potential of the squid axon revealed that 1.0 mM of RAC 109 I caused an 88 per cent reduction in the maximum rate of depolarization following internal perfusion, while the same concentration of RAC 109 II produced only a 53 per cent decrease in the maximum rate of depolarization. Subsequent voltage clamp studies on the frog sciatic nerve demonstrated a 76 per cent reduction in sodium conductance following application of 0.28 nM of RAC 109 I, but only a 42–57 per cent decrease in sodium permeability when RAC 109 II was used. Thus, RAC 109 II was approximately 20–60 per cent more active than RAC 109 I in terms of decreasing the rate of depolarization and sodium conductance. In addition, the minimum concentration (Cm) of RAC 109 II required for conduction blockade in sheathed frog sciatic nerve was five times less than that of RAC 109 I. In the desheathed preparation a 3-fold difference in Cm existed between the two isomers. Although these results are suggestive of a stereospecific local anaesthetic receptor, the possibility remains that the difference in activity between isomers might be related to differential uptake and penetration of the membrane. This possibility was evaluated by Akerman[18] in several ways. The uptake of radioactive RAC 109 I and II by both sheathed and desheathed frog sciatic nerves was measured and no difference was observed in the uptake of the two isomers by the isolated sciatic nerve. Additional studies also failed to reveal any difference between the uptake and binding of radioactive RAC 109 I and II to erythrocyte and synaptosome membranes or to the phospolipid, phosphatidyl-serine, which is known to be a component of nerve membrane. Since the isomers of RAC 109 penetrate membranes to the same extent, possess similar physico-chemical properties and similar proportions of charged and uncharged form, their differential anaesthetic potencies would be difficult to explain in terms of the surface charge theory, or change in membrane volume, or configuration hypothesis. The action of the optical isomers of RAC 109 are consistent with the concept of differential binding to stereospecific receptors located within the sodium channel.

Selectivity of binding of tetrodotoxin and saxitoxin

Several naturally occurring biotoxins, saxitoxin and tetrodotoxin, exist which are capable of producing profound conduction blockade in isolated nerves. These substances are unique biologically, since they act specifically on the sodium channel to inhibit sodium conductance. Their site of action appears to be located on the external surface of the sodium channel, since internal and external perfusion of the giant squid axon with solutions of tetrodotoxin revealed that external perfusion with 1×10^{-7} M resulted in inhibition of a propagated action potential within 3–6 minutes.[19] On the other hand, axoplasmic perfusion with 1×10^{-6} M and 1×10^{-5} M tetrodotoxin for as long as 17–37 minutes had no effect on the maximum rate of rise of the action potential. Moreover, Colquhoun and Ritchie[20] and Henderson, Ritchie and Strichartz[21] have shown that conventional local anaesthetics such as lignocaine do not alter the binding of the biotoxins to the membrane.

A competitive antagonism does exist between TTX and STX. Henderson, Ritchie and Strichartz demonstrated that the specific binding of 4 nM of STX to frog myelinated fibers was reduced by 95 per cent when 500 nM of TTX was added to the perfusion medium.[21] Divalent ions such as calcium, which are believed to act at the external surface of the nerve membrane, are also capable of displacing TTX and STX from membrane binding sites. For example, in the absence of calcium, 100 per cent of TTX and STX are bound to solubilized garfish membrane preparations. In the presence of 50 mM of calcium, only 28 per cent of TTX and 34 per cent STX were bound to the garfish membrane preparation.

The binding of the biotoxins to the external opening of the sodium channel is so specific that these agents have been utilized to determine the size and number of sodium channels in various nerve preparations. Hille[22] has calculated that the external opening of the sodium channel is a space 3 Å wide by 5 Å long lined by six oxygen atoms. One molecule of TTX or STX will occupy one sodium channel opening. On the basis of the studies with TTX and STX, it was concluded that approximately 30 sodium channels/cm^2 exist in the rabbit vagus nerve, whereas in the unmyelinated fibres of the garfish olfactory nerve, there are only 6 sodium channels/cm^2. However, studies utilizing an improved method for labeling STX indicated a significantly greater density of sodium channels. Data presented by Ritchie, Rogart and Strichartz[23] based on STX binding sites calculated 110 sodium channels/cm^2 in garfish nerves. In summary, the investigations with the biotoxins provide additional evidence that the basic mechanism of local anaesthesia involves combination with a specific membrane receptor which is located at the external opening of the sodium channel.

Frequency-dependent conduction blockade
A number of studies have been conducted which show that the effect of local anaesthetics on the sodium conductance and action potential of nerves is influenced by the rate of stimulation of a nerve at the time of local anaesthetic application (Fig. 2.6). Strichartz[24] demonstrated that the quaternary derivative of lignocaine, QX-314, could inhibit sodium currents

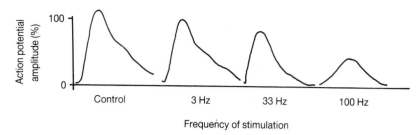

Figure 2.6   Effect of stimulation frequency on local anaesthetic induced conduction block.

by more than 90 per cent following axoplasmic perfusion of the frog sciatic nerve. Application of depolarizing pulses of 5 ms duration at 1 s. intervals enhanced the rate and degree of sodium permeability inhibition produced by QX-314. This phenomenon has been referred to as 'use dependent inhibition'. An increase in frequency of stimulation without a local anaesthetic does not effect the sodium currents. In the absence of depolarizing pulses, QX-314 requires 20–30 minutes to produce maximum inhibition of sodium permeability. A combination of internal perfusion of the membrane with QX-314 and application of 20 depolarizing pulses caused maximal inhibition of sodium permeability within 5 minutes. In addition, a direct correlation exists between the frequency of nerve stimulation and the degree of sodium conductance blockade.

These studies with QX-314 also suggest that the receptor site for conventional local anaesthetics is located close to the internal opening of the sodium channel. Axoplasmic perfusion with QX-314 resulted in rapid conduction blockade while application of this charged local anaesthetic to the external surface of the nerve membrane caused minimal effects on sodium currents.

Courtney[25] has also evaluated frequency-dependent conduction blockade with a tertiary amine-type of local anaesthetic agent. Most of the experiments were performed with an experimental tertiary amine compound, GEA 968, which is structurally related to lignocaine. Again, a direct correlation was found between the frequency of stimulation and the degree of inhibition of inward sodium currents in myelinated frog nerves. In the presence of 0.5 mM of GEA 968, repetitive depolarization at the rate of 2 pulses/s. resulted in a progressive decrease in sodium conductance, such that inward sodium current was decreased by 76 per cent after 25 pulses. Similar frequency-dependent inhibition of sodium permeability was observed with procaine and lignocaine, although frequencies of at least 2 pulses/s. were required to clearly demonstrate this relationship with the latter.

Following maximal depression of sodium permeability and a period of rest, the inhibitory effect of both tertiary amine and quaternary-type local anaesthetics can be reversed by an increase in the frequency of nerve stimulation. Under conditions in which a large hyperpolarizing prepulse is applied to the nerve followed by a series of depolarizing pulses, the rate of reversal of local anaesthetic activity is directly related to the frequency of stimulation.

This phenomenon of use or frequency-dependent inhibition has been interpreted in the following manner. At rest, sodium channels are closed which prevents sodium flux across the membrane. During nerve stimulation, the sodium channels assume the open state to allow the influx of sodium ions which is essential for membrane depolarization. An increase in the frequency of stimulation will permit the sodium channels to remain in an open state for a longer period of time. In addition, the degree of depolarization pulses will determine the number of channels that are open. The size and number of depolarizing pulses basically effect the phase of sodium activation. Application of a hyperpolarizing prepulse to the membrane is believed to prevent the phase of sodium inactivation. Thus, the combination of a hyperpolarizing prepulse and a series of depolarizing pulses of optimal size will maximize the number and duration of sodium channels opened. Both tertiary and quarternary local anaesthetic activity is enhanced. The onset of conduction block is decreased and the duration of blockade is shortened when the gates of the sodium channels are open. This strongly supports the concept that a specific local anaesthetic receptor is located within the sodium channel which is readily accessible when sodium channels are in the open position.

Multiple versus single site of anaesthetic action

On the basis of studies with various substances that can produce conduction blockade in peripheral nerve, two theories have currently evolved concerning the site of action of local anaesthetic agents. One theory suggests that various sites of action exist for conduction blocking agents of different chemical types. The following classification summarizes the different sites of action that may exist in the nerve membrane.

(A)   External surface of the sodium channel. The biotoxin substances, tetrodotoxin and saxitoxin are believed to act at this location.

(B)   The axoplasmic side of the sodium channel. The quaternary derivatives of lignocaine such as QX-314, QX-572 and QX-222 act at this site.

(C)   Within the nerve membrane causing an expansion of the membrane or a change in membrane configuration. Agents such as benzocaine, n-butanol and benzyl alcohol, i.e. the neutral-type of local anaesthetic drugs are believed to cause conduction block in this fashion.

(D)   Site of action both at the axoplasmic side of the sodium channel and also within the membrane. Most of the clinically useful local anaesthetic agents, since they exist both in charged and uncharged form, e.g. procaine, amethocaine, lignocaine, mepivacaine, prilocaine, bupivacaine and etidocaine are believed to act at these sites. The cationic form of these drugs would interact with a specific receptor in the axoplasmic portion of the sodium channel while the uncharged base form would act by a physico-chemical mechanism within the membrane. Narahashi and Frazier[26] have suggested that approximately 90 per cent of the blocking action of an agent such as lignocaine is referable to its cationic form and 10 per cent is due to the base form.

Hille[2] has attempted to provide a unified theory for the site of action of both charged and uncharged forms of local anaesthetic drugs. A voltage clamp technique was employed to study the action of tertiary amine, quaternary amine and neutral type local anaesthetics on sodium conductance in myelinated fibers of the isolated frog sciatic nerve. Hille's theory was based on a re-evaluation of the relationship between lipid solubility, pH, voltage and frequency-dependent modulation and the rate, degree and reversal of local anaesthetic depression of sodium permeability. The time required to block half of the sodium currents varied as a function of the pK_a and the lipid solubility of the compounds and the pH of the bathing solution. In general, low pK_a and high lipid solubility and pH enhanced the onset of blockade. The results again demonstrated that the onset of action of neutral and charged agents is pH independent and the quaternary amine agents which exist only in the charged form are relatively inactive when applied to the external surface of the nerve. In addition, tertiary amine and quaternary amine molecules demonstrate voltage and frequency-dependent inhibition, but the neutral agent, benzocaine, did not show a similar effect.

The model proposed involves a single receptor in the sodium channel for neutral, tertiary and quaternary types of local anaesthetics. However, differences do exist in the pathways which these various substances use to reach the receptor site. The hydrophilic quaternary amine compounds such as QX-314, are unable to penetrate the lipid-rich membrane. Thus, these agents can only reach the receptor site from the internal aqueous medium when the sodium channels are open. The neutral lipophilic agents such as benzocaine penetrate into the core of the lipid membrane and use a hydrophobic pathway to reach the receptor site even when sodium channels are in the closed or inactive state (Fig. 2.7). Since tertiary amines such as procaine and lignocaine exist both in a charged hydrophilic and uncharged lipophilic form, they may reach the receptor site by both the hydrophilic and hydrophobic pathways. The uncharged base utilizes the hydrophobic path and so can reach the receptor site while the sodium channel is in the closed or inactivated state. The cationic form must use the hydrophilic pathway and so can only reach the receptor when the sodium channels are open (Fig. 2.7). Hille's hypothesis does not account for the action of the biotoxins at the external surface of the sodium channel. However, the chemical configuration of the biotoxins is sufficiently different from other types of local anaesthetic agents that they may be unable to enter the inner

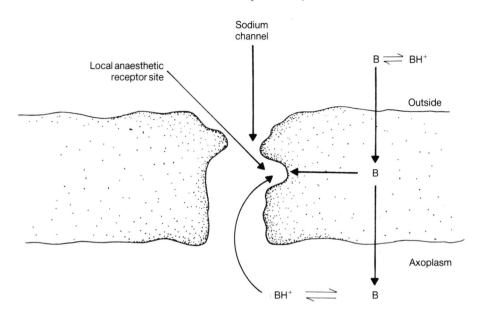

Figure 2.7 Mechanism of local anaesthetic induced conduction block.

aperture of the sodium channel even when the gates are open, but may be able to reach the local anaesthetic receptor from the external surface of the sodium channel.

Butterworth and coworkers[27] have attempted to determine the depth of the local anaesthetic binding site within the nerve membrane. Biotin containing polyethylene glycols of zero, three and six ethylene glycol subunits were attached to the p-amino end of amethocaine and procaine. Thus, compounds of various lengths were synthesized which contained the active anaesthetic end, a pharmacologically inert chain of varying length and the inactive biotin on the opposite end. These derivatives of procaine and amethocaine produced both tonic and use-dependent blockade of desheathed frog sciatic nerves in a concentration-dependent fashion. When avidin, a high molecular weight protein that binds to biotin, was added to the solution bathing the isolated nerve, no conduction block was produced by the procaine and amethocaine derivatives. Presumably the avidin was bound to the biotin end of the molecules and thus restricted the biotin to the external surface of the nerve membrane. Apparently, the length of the local anaesthetic derivatives was too short to allow the active end to reach the site of action in the sodium channel. Since the largest agent that contained six ethylene glycol units places the active end of the molecule 15–19 Å from the surface of the nerve membrane, it was concluded that the local anaesthetic receptor site must be located at a distance greater than 15–18 Å from the external surface of the nerve membrane.

Active form of conventional local anaesthetics

In solution, the clinically useful local anaesthetic agents exist both in the form of uncharged molecules (B) and as positively charged cations (BH⁺). The relative proportion between the uncharged base (B) and the charged cation (BH⁺) is dependent on the pH of the solution and pK_a of the specific chemical compound and can be determined by the Henderson–Hasselbalch equation:

$$pH = pK_a - \log (B)/(BH^+)$$

Since pK_a is constant for any specific compound the relative proportion of free base and charged cation in a local anaesthetic solution is basically dependent on the pH of the solution. As the pH of the solution is decreased and hydrogen ion concentration is increased, more of the local anaesthetic will exist in the charged cationic form. Conversely, an increase in pH and decrease in hydrogen ions will result in the formation of relatively greater amounts of the free base form. Ritchie, Ritchie and Greengard[28],[29] conducted a series of experiments which evaluated the relationship between the pH of solutions of lignocaine and cinchocaine and local anaesthetic activity in isolated sheath and desheathed nerves. When isolated nerves possessing an intact sheath were used, it was found that as the pH of the bathing solution containing either lignocaine or cinchocaine was raised from 7.2 to 9.2, the rate of reduction in the height of the surface action potential was markedly increased.

Thus, alkaline solutions containing relatively greater amounts of the uncharged base (B) were more active in suppressing electrical activity of the sheathed nerve. However, when the experiments were repeated with a desheathed nerve preparation, the results differed. At a pH of 7.2, cinchocaine (10 uM) produced a 90 per cent reduction in spike potential amplitude, whereas only 10 per cent depression in spike potential occurred when the pH was elevated to 9.2. Similarly, 300 uM of lignocaine produced almost complete abolishment of the spike potential at a pH of 7.2. In an alkaline solution (pH = 9.2–10.7), the same concentration of lignocaine resulted in only a 50 per cent decrease in action potential amplitude. Under these experimental conditions, the less alkaline local anaesthetic solution, which would contain a relatively greater amount of the charged cation (BH+), was more active in terms of conduction blockade. Additional evidence favouring the cationic moiety as the active form of local anaesthetics was forthcoming from experiments by Narahashi, Yamada and Frazier[30],[31] who studied the conduction blocking properties of two tertiary and two quaternary derivatives of lignocaine. The tertiary amine derivatives can exist partially in a charged and uncharged form, whereas the quarternary compounds possess only a charged configuration. When tertiary amine derivatives can exist partially in a charged and uncharged form, whereas the quarternary compounds possess only a charged configuration. When the tertiary amine compounds were applied to the external surface of the axon, a 13 per cent decrease in the maximum rate of rise of the action potential (dV/dt) was observed. Increasing the pH from 7.0 to 9.0 did not effect the degree of reduction in dV/dt. Internal perfusion of the tertiary amine at a pH of 7.0 caused a 57 per cent decrease in dV/dt. However, only a 20 per cent reduction in dV/dt occurred when the pH of the internal perfusion medium was elevated to 8.0. Since the increase in pH would tend to lower the relative concentration of the cationic form of the local anaesthetic, these results again demonstrate that the charged moiety is primarily responsible for conduction blockade. However, tertiary amines are capable of diffusion across membranes so that they are effective conduction blockers following either external or internal application. In order to overcome the problem of diffusion, quaternary derivatives of lignocaine were utilized. These compounds exist only as cations, which do not diffuse readily across membranes. External application of 10 mM of the quaternary compound, QX-314, produced less than a 10 per cent decrease in dV/dt in the squid axon. Internal perfusion of 1 mM of QX-314 caused a mean reduction of 67 per cent in dV/dt. Strichartz[24] extended these studies by determining the effects of the quaternary derivatives of lignocaine on sodium permeability of the frog sciatic nerve. External application of 5 mM of QX-314 decreased the amplitude of the inward sodium currents by 7 per cent. By contrast, internal application of only 0.5 mM of QX-314 diminished the sodium currents by almost 90 per cent. Since all the above studies were carried out with lignocaine and its derivatives, Narahashi and Frazier investigated the effects of internal and external perfusion of procaine at different pH levels on the sodium permeability of the squid axon. The results demonstrated that procaine also acts primarily in the cationic form at the internal opening of the sodium channel.

On the basis of these observations, it has been postulated that the uncharged base form of local anaesthetics is responsible for optimal diffusion through the nerve sheath. After penetration of the nerve sheath and the nerve membrane, re-equilibrium occurs between the base and cationic form in the axoplasm and the charged cationic form of the drug then diffuses to the receptor site within the sodium channel. The attachment of the cationic form of the local anaesthetic to the receptor in the sodium channel results in a decrease in sodium conductance which, in turn, causes conduction blockade.

Differential nerve blockade

Classically, the susceptibility of nerves to conduction blockade was considered to be related to the fibre size, i.e. a greater concentration of local anaesthetic agent is required to block nerves of large diameter. This relationship between fibre size and anaesthetic sensitivity in myelinated nerves was believed to be a function of the length of the nerve fibre and number of nodes exposed to the local anaesthetic solution. It was originally reported that three consecutive nodes must be inactivated by a high concentration of local anaesthetic agent in order to produce complete conduction block in a myelinated nerve.[32] Since the distance between successive nodes is greater in large myelinated fibres than in small diameter fibres, Franz and Perry[33] postulated that differential blockade of myelinated fibres was due primarily to diffusion of local anaesthetic along the nerve fibres. Small fibres would be blocked due to the short internodal distance while larger fibres would not be completely blocked since the local anaesthetic would not diffuse a sufficient distance to inactivate three consecutive nodes.

More recently Fink and Cairns[34] failed to observe a size-related differential sensitivity to equilibrium conduction block in mammaliam myelinated fibres exposed to lignocaine. At high concentrations of local anaesthetic no difference in nodal sensitivity to conduction block was observed in large and small myelinated fibres. Thus, sensitivity to conduction block based on fibre size cannot explain the clinical observations of differential nerve blockade. However, when minimum effective concentrations (ED_{50}) of local anaesthetic are employed, differential block may occur provided that a sufficient length of nerve is exposed to the local anaesthetic. Fink and Cairns[34] suggest that at low local anaesthetic concentrations, the probability of blocking three consecutive nodes is decreased due to a variety of factors. An increase in the length of the nerve exposed to a sufficient volume of dilute local anaesthetic solution should enhance the probability of inactivating three consecutive nodes and so inducing complete conduction block.

A possible explanation for this relationship between length of nerve exposed to low local anaesthetic concentrations and incidence of conduction block has been provided by Raymond and coworkers.[35] These authors demonstrated that the concentration of local anaesthetic required for 50 per cent of impulses in single myelinated fibres diminished as the exposed length of the nerve increased. These results are believed related to decremental conduction, i.e. a partial inactivation of the nodes exposed to low concentration of local anaesthetic extends the decay of the action potential along the axon. If the length of axon is sufficiently long, and conduction block will ultimately occur. These data do not support the original assumption that the length of the nerve beyond three nodes is not a factor in conduction block. This concept of decremental conduction, which was originally described by Lorente de No and Condouris,[36] provides an alternative explanation for differential conduction blockade. Fink[37] has employed this concept of decremental conduction to explain the phenomenon of differential spinal block.

The relative sensitivity of myelinated and unmyelinated fibres to local anaesthetic induced conduction block has also been reinvestigated. The classic study of Gasser and Erlanger[38] has led mistakenly to the conclusion that small myelinated fibres are intrinsically more sensitive to local anaesthetic induced conduction block than large myelinated fibres. Condouris, Goebel and Brady[39] used a computer simulation of local anaesthetic blockade to study the characteristics of blockade produced by TTX and lignocaine. This model predicted that myelinated nerves were more susceptible to local anaesthetic blockade than unmyelinated fibres. Gissen, Covino and Gregus[40, 42] re-evaluated the Cm of various local anaesthetics in mammalian myelinated and unmyelinated fibres. The Cm of lignocaine, amethocaine, etidocaine and bupivacaine required to produce a 50 per cent decrease in the amplitude of the action potential of myelinated fibres from the desheathed rabbit vagus nerve was significantly less than the Cm required for unmyelinated C fibres (Fig. 2.8). These *in vitro* results appear to differ from *in vivo* clinical studies in which low concentrations of local anaesthetic produce exclusively sensory blockade indicating inactivation of small unmyelinated C fibres only. As the concentration is increased, inhibition of small myelinated B fibres and finally motor blockade (inhibition of large myelinated A fibres) can be achieved. Gissen, Covino and Gregus[41, 42] have attempted to explain these apparently conflicting results as follows: in isolated nerves exposed to low concentrations of local anaesthetics, a reduction in the action potential amplitude of C fibres is initially observed. However, with time, the action potential of A fibres begins to show suppression and ultimately the degree of A fibre action potential

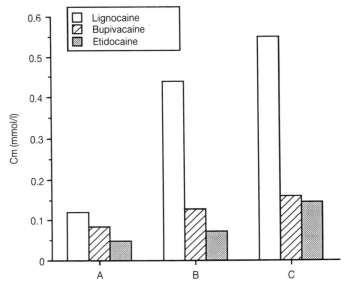

Figure 2.8 Minimum concentration of various local anesthetics required for 50 per cent reduction in action potential amplitude of A, B and C fibres.

depression exceeds that of the C fibres indicating that at equilibrium the Cm for A fibres is less than that of C fibres. However, in an *in vitro* situation the isolated nerve is devoid of circulation such that the local anaesthetic remains in continuous contact with the nerve fibres. In an *in vivo* situation with intact circulation, some of the local anaesthetic injected in the region of a peripheral nerve will diffuse to the nerve membrane while some of the local anaesthetic will be absorbed by the vascular system and carried away from the site of injection. Thus, following injection of a low concentration of local anaesthetic in an intact animal a sufficient amount of the drug may penetrate to the non-myelinated C fibres which do not have many diffusion barriers and cause conduction block of these sensory fibers. However, the large myelinated fibres are protected by diffusion barriers such that, as the local anaesthetic slowly penetrates to the nerve membrane of the A fibers, it is also being absorbed by the vascular system resulting in a significant decrease in the amount of drug which ultimately will reach the receptor site at the nerve membrane. If the absorption of local anaesthetic is sufficient to reduce the concentration of drug arriving at the nerve membrane of the A fiber to below the Cm for that particular fibre, conduction block will not occur. Under these conditions it is possible to achieve differential sensory block without significant motor blockade.

In summary, recent neurophysiological studies indicate that the safety margin for conduction blockade is less in large A fibres than small C fibres following exposure of isolated nerves to local anaesthetics. However, differential sensory/motor blockade is still possible in clinical situations due to differences in the diffusional barriers surrounding A and C fibres and the absorption of injected local anaesthetics by the vascular system.

References

1. Chiu, S. Y. and Ritchie, J. M. Potassium channels in nodal and internodal axonal membrane of mammalian myelinated fibers. *Nature* 1980 **284**: 170–1
2. Hille, B. *Ionic Channels of Excitable Membranes.* Sunderland, Mass: Sinauer Associates 1984.
3. Aceves, J., and Machne, X. The action of calcium and local anaesthetics on nerve cells and their interaction during excitation. *Pharmacol. Exp. Ther.* **140**: 138–48.
4. Shanes, A. M., Freygang, W. H., Grundgest, H., and Amatniek, E. Anesthetic and Calcium Action in the Voltage Clamped Squid Giant Axon. *J. Gen. Physio.* **42**: 793–802.
5. Condouris, G. A. A Study of the mechanism of action of cocaine on amphibian peripheral nerve. *J. Pharmacol. Exp. Thera.* 1961; **1312**: 243–9.
6. Taylor, R. E. Effect of Procaine on Electrical Properties of Squid Axon Membrane. *Amer. J. Physiol.* 1959; **196**: 1071–8.
7. Hille, B. The common mode of action of three agents that decrease the

transient charge in sodium permeability in nerves. *Nature* 1966; **210**: 1220–2.

8. Strichartz, G. Inhibition of tonic currents in myelinated nerves by quaternary derivatives of lidocaine. *Mol. Mech. Anesth.* 1975; **1**: 1–11.

9. Hille, B. Pharmacological modifications of the sodium channels of frog nerve. *J. Gen. Physiol.* 1968; **51**: 199–219.

10. Frazier, D. T., Narahashi, T., and Yamada, M. The site of action and active form of local anaesthetics. II. Experiments with quaternary compounds. *J. Pharmacol. Exp. Thera.* 1970; **171**: 45–51.

11. Seeman, P. The Membrane Action of Anaesthetics and Tranquilizers. *Pharmacol. Rev.* 1972; **24**: 583–655.

12 Skou, J. C. Local anaesthetics. VI. Relation between blocking potency and penetration of a monomolecular layer of lipoids from nerves. *Acta Pharmacol. Toxicol.* 1954; **10**: 325–37.

13. Roth, S. H., Smith R. A., and Paton, D. M. Pressure antagonism of anaesthesia-induced conduction failure in frog peripheral nerve. *Brit. J. Anaesth.* 1976; **48**: 621–8.

14. Kendig, J. J., and Cohen, E. N. Pressure antagonism to nerve conduction block by anaesthetic agents. *Anesthesiology* 1977; **47**: 6–10.

15. Boggs, J. M., Roth, S. H., Yoong, T., Wong, E., and Hsia, J. C. Site and mechanism of anaesthetic action. II. pressure effect on the nerve conducting-blocking activity of a spin-label anaesthetic. *Mol. Pharmacol.* 1976; **12**: 136–43.

16. Singer S. J., and Nicholson, G. L. Thew Fluid Mosaic Model of the Structure of Cell Membranes. *Scienced* 1972; **175**: 720–31.

17. Feinstein, M. B. Reaction of local anaesthetics with phospholipids. A possible Chemical Basis of Anaesthesia. *J. Gen. Physiol.* 1964; **48**: 357–74.

18. Akerman, B. *Studies on the Relative Pharmacological Effects of Enantiomers of Local Anaesthetics with Special Regard to Block of Nervous Excitation.* Doctoral Dissertation. 1973; Sweden. Uppsala.

19. Narahashiu, T., Anderson, N. C., and Moore, J. W. Comparison of tetrodotoxin and procaine in internally perfused squid giant axons. *J. Gen. Physiol.* 1967; **50**: 1413–28.

20 Colquhoun, D. and Ritchie, J. M. The interaction at equilibration between tetrodotoxin and mammalian non-myelinated nerve fibers. *J. Physiol.* 1972; **221**: 533–53.

21 Henderson, R., Ritchie, J, M., and Strichartz, G. R. The binding of labelled saxitoxin to the sodium channels in nerve membranes. *J. Physiol.* 1973; **235**: 783–804.

22. Hille, B. The permeability of the sodium channel to organic cations in myelinated nerve. *J. Gen. Physiol.* 1971; **58**: 599–619.

23. Ritchie, J. M., Rogart, R. B., and Strichartz, G. R. A new method for labelling saxitoxin and its binding to non-myelinated fibers of the rabbit vagus, lobster walking leg and garfish olfactory nerves. *J. Physiol.* 1976; **261**: 477–94.

24 Strichartz, G. R. The inhibition of sodium currents in myelinated nerve by quaternary derivatives of lidocaine. *J. Gen. Physiol.* 1973; **62**: 37–57.

25 Courtney, K. R. Mechanisms of frequency-dependent inhibition of sodium currents in frog myelinated nerve by the lidocaine derivative GEA 968. *J. Pharmacol. Exp. Ther.* 1975; **195**: 225–36.

26   Narahashi, T., and Frazier, D. T., Site of action and active form of local anesthetics. *Neurosci. Res. Program Bull* 1971; **4**: 65-99.

27   Butterworth, J. F., Moran, J. R., Whitesides, G. M., and Strichartz, G. R. Limited nerve impulse blockade by 'Leashed' local anesthetics. *J. Med. Chem.* 1987; **30**: 1295–302.

28   Ritchie, J. M., Ritchie, B., and Greengard, P. The active structure of local anesthetics. *J. Pharmacol. Exp. Thera.* 1965; **150**: 152–9.

29   Ritchie, J. M., Ritchie, B., and Greengard, P. The effect of the nerve sheath on the action of local anesthetics. *J. Pharmacol. Exp. Thera.* 1965; **150**: 160–4.

30. Narahashi, T., Yamada, M., and Frazier, D. T. Cationic forms of local anesthetics block action potentials from inside the nerve membrane. *Nature.* 1969; **223**: 748–9.

31   Narahashi, T., Frazier, D., and Yamada, M. The site of action and active form of local anesthetics. I. Theory and pH experiments with tertiary compounds. *J. Pharmacol. Exp. Thera.* 1970; **171**: 32–44.

32. Tasaki, I. *Nervous Transmissions.* Springfield, Mass. Thomas, 1953.

33. Franz, D. N. and Perry, R. S. Mechanism for differential block among single myelinated and non-myelinated axons by procaine. *J. Physiol. (London)* 1979; **236**: 193–210.

34. Fink, B. R. and Cairns, A. M. Lack of size-related differential sensitivity to equilibrium conduction block among mammalian myelinated fibers with Lidocaine. *Anesthesia and Analgesia* 1987; **66**: 948–53.

35   Raymond, S. A., Steffensen, S. C., Gugino, L. D., and Strichartz, G. R. The role of length of nerve exposed to local anesthetics in impulse blocking action. *Anesthesia and Analgesia* 1989; **68**: 563–70.

36. Lorente de No, R. and Cond#uris, G. Decremental Conductions in Peripheral Nerve Integration of Stimuli in the Neuron. *Proc. Nat. Acad. Sci. (USA)* 1959; **45**: 592–617.

37. Fink, B. R. Mechanisms of differential axial blockade in epidural and subarachnoid anesthesia. *Anesthesiology* 1989; **70**: 851–8.

38. Gasser H. B. and Erlanger, J. The Role of Fiber size in the establishment of a nerve block by pressure or cocaine. *Amer. J. Physiol.* 1929; **88**: 581–91.

39. Condouris, G. A., Goebel, R. H. and Brady T. Computer simulation of local anesthetic effects using a mathematical model of myelinated nerve. *J. Pharmacol. Exp. Thera.* 1976; **196**: 737–45.

40. Gissen, A. J., Covino, B. G., and Gregus, J. Differential sensitivies of mammalian nerve fibers to local anesthestic agents. *Anesthesiology* 1980; **53**: 467–74.

41. Gissen, A. J., Covino, B. G., and Gregus, J. Differential sensitivity of fast and slow fibers in mammalian nerve. II. Margin of safety for nerve transmission. *Anesthesia and Analgesia* 1982; **61**: 561–9.

42. Gissen, A. J., Covino, B. G., and Gregus, J. Differential sensitivity of fast and slow fibers in mammalian nerve. III. Effect of etidocaine and bupivacaine on fast and slow fibers. *Anesthesia and Analgesia* 1982; **61**: 570–5.

3

Mechanisms of transmitter block

K. Budd
R. G. Hill

Introduction

Pain is the cogniscent counterpart of the body's response to breaches of its integrity. The aversive nature of pain strongly motivates the organism to avoid continuing threatening situations and this avoidance of contact or mobility of a damaged area may aid in the healing process. However, pain may continue beyond this period of useful purpose and result in profound behavioural changes and physical suffering as a response to a complex interaction of motor, sensory, autonomic and psychological factors. The manner in which the impingement of a noxious stimulus on to the organism is converted to the sensory experience is highly complex and subject to many modulatory influences between origin and cortical appreciation. There are, however, neural circuits within which afferent fibres and neurons can be identified as responding to noxious stimuli and can, therefore, be presumed to be involved in the transference of pain.

Anatomically distinct pain receptors as such have not been identified and it is presumed that the free, unmyelinated nerve endings found ubiquitously in dermal and epidermal layers, muscles and viscera, subserve this function. Pain is transmitted from these free endings by an incompletely understood transduction process leading to the generation of action potentials in the small sensory nerve fibres. The first synapses occur within the dorsal horn of the spinal cord and it is possible to influence the onward transmission of action potentials at various points along sensory nerve fibres by the use of drugs, which may be administered locally or systematically, or the use of a variety of physical manoeuvres. It must be remembered, however, that the sensory, afferent nerves are not the only nervous structures amenable to blockade for diagnostic and therapeutic purposes. The autonomic nervous system is frequently involved in painful pathologies and blockade of this essentially efferent system is of great importance in the confirmation of the diagnosis of autonomically mediated or maintained pain and its therapy.

It is difficult to make a clear distinction between efferent and afferent fibres however, for many of the internal organs have not only a dual sympathetic and parasympathetic innervation but sensory afferent fibres usually run with both sets of these nerves. For most abdominal structures and for the heart and lower part of the oesophagus nociceptive responses can be attributed entirely to afferents that run in autonomic nerves largely of the sympathetic division.[1] However, nociceptive afferents running with parasympathetic nerves exist for the airways leading to and within the lungs and for some of the pelvic organs. To further complicate matters, many afferents running in sympathetic nerves are clearly not exclusively nociceptive since they respond strongly to stimuli within the normal range of physiological activity.[2] Thus it can be seen that the peripheral nervous system mirrors the complexity of the central organization and that a simplistic view of function and response is of little value when planning diagnostic and therapeutic strategies.

Tissue damage and mediator release

Although differences have been described across species, it is generally observed that in mammalian skin, and in most other tissues, two distinct classes of nociceptive afferent unit occur. These are high threshold mechanoreceptors with A-delta axons (HTM) and polymodal nociceptors with C axons (PMN).[3, 4] Both HTM and PMN have small receptive fields. Whilst the former appear specialized for detecting mechanical stresses in the damaging range, the latter also respond to strong mechanical stimuli but in addition show a sensitivity to the chemicals released in damaged or inflamed skin, thus signalling the presence of these agents. The sensitivity of all classes of nociceptor increases following mild injury and this results in hyperalgesia in injured tissues. Damage may directly excite nerve endings by mechanical, thermal or chemical effects on the membrane. This damage also initiates a sequence of events appreciated as inflammation with pain as one of its major characteristics. Release of chemical agents will initiate or mediate this response and among those implicated are the substances listed in Table 3.1.[5] Although not strictly correct, these algogenic substances will be included within the definition of transmitter for the purposes of this chapter.

C fibre afferents are characteristically known to contain peptides, including substance P, somatostatin, cholecystokinin, calcitonin gene related peptide (CGRP), vasoactive intestinal peptide, and (in rodents) sometimes contain the enzyme fluoride resistant acid phosphatase. The co-existence of any two of these agents in the same fibres does not exclude

Table 3.1   Pain producing substances and potentiators

Hydrogen ions
Potassium ions
Acetylcholine
Histamine
Bradykinin
Serotonin
Adenosine triphosphate
Prostaglandins

the possibility of functions other than the transmitting of information by coded nerve impulses.[6] There is good evidence that C fibres also play a role in the periphery by way of the axon reflex which produces three local reactions to injury – vasodilatation (flare), neurogenic oedema (wheal) and sensitization of nerve endings.[7] This is likely to be due to the release of substance P and other peptides from the nerve, indirectly provoking the release of a number of other substances including histamine from mast cells.[8] Histamine increases skin blood flow and can produce a sensation of itch, but does not usually give rise to intense pain. Bradykinin and 5-hydroxytryptamine are, however, powerful stimulants of peripheral nociceptors having little effect upon other sensory receptors and both are released by tissue injury.[9] Neurophysiological evidence suggests that bradykinin is an important mediator of pain and hyperalgesia in inflammatory reactions[10] and that it is also capable of stimulating the synthesis and release of prostaglandins by the activation of phospholipase A_2.[12] It has also been proposed that the pain and hyperalgesia associated with inflammation is, at least in part, dependent upon the potentiation of the effects of 5-hydroxytryptamine and the kinins by prostaglandins.[11] Direct tissue damage will also release prostaglandins, which will sensitize the nociceptors to the action of bradykinin. In addition to the prostaglandins, lipoxygenase products will also sensitize nociceptors and the most potent agent is likely to be 8 (R), 15 (S) di-HETE.[13] Cytokines are also released into damaged tissues and interleukin–1–β has been shown to be a potent hyperalgesic agent in animal studies. This action does not seem to be dependent on PG release as it is still seen in animals treated with indomethacin.[14]

Clinically, most relevant pain states build up slowly and outlast the precipitating cause. In such cases, the protective nature of pain may change from the initiation of escape to the generation of processes that aid recovery and repair. There would appear to be a novel group of nociceptors particularly responsive to these slow changes in the state of inflamed peripheral tissue whilst being unaffected by transient excessive mechanical or thermal stimuli. The presence of these 'silent' nociceptors (primary afferent fibres that do not respond to acute noxious mechanical or thermal stimuli) has only recently become apparent with the discovery of mechanically and thermally insensitive cutaneous afferent C fibres, at least some of which are excited by irritant chemicals or are recruited during inflammatory states.[15] The activation of these afferents in chronically inflamed or injured tissue may not only represent an extra source of nociceptive input, but may also be important in promoting changes in the central nervous system. This may include slowly developing, but maintained, central sensitization in which dorsal horn cells show enhanced ongoing activity and responsiveness to peripheral stimulation and sometimes increases in receptive field size. Such changes in central excitability are triggered by activity in primary afferent C fibres that are highly likely to be of the 'silent' variety.

The mechanisms by which the constituent transmitters of C fibres promote nociception are complex. These pseudo-monopolar fibres release their transmitters both from their peripheral terminals (as described above in the context of the axon reflex) and from their central terminals within the dorsal horn of the spinal cord, where the consequence is excitation of relay neurones whose axons project to higher levels of the central nervous system. It is therefore likely that drugs which interfere with the action of C-fibre transmitters will have a component of their action in the periphery and a component within the spinal cord, unless pharmacokinetic factors exclude the drug in question from the central nervous system.

Pharmacotherapy

Histamine

The use of antihistamines in treating pain is somewhat contentious. Any beneficial selective effects of histamine receptor blockers are confined to antagonism of responses to the histamine that is released.

Although most H_1 blockers have a local anaesthetic effect, this probably does not entirely account for their marked degree of success in countering the stimulant action of histamine on nerve endings. There is little correlation between the local anaesthetic potency of these drugs and their ability to inhibit neural responses to histamine. The local anaesthetic effect of antihistamines is variable, some being more potent than procaine, (e.g. promethazine and pyrillamine), but the concentrations required to produce this effect are several orders of magnitude higher than those needed to antagonize the effects of histamine.[16] Like histamine itself most antihistamines active at the H_1 receptor contain a substituted ethylamine moiety, but unlike histamine, which has a primary amino group and a single aromatic ring, most H_1 blockers have a tertiary amino group linked by a two- or three- atom chain to two aromatic substituents.[17] The different classes of H_1 blocking drugs are shown in Table 3.2. All of these agents have the facility for systemic or topical application and, to a large extent, share similar side effect profiles.

Table 3.2 H_1 receptor antagonist drugs

1. Ethanolamines e.g. diphenhydramine.
2. Ethylenediamines e.g. pyrillamine.
3. Alkyalamines e.g. chlorpheniramine.
4. Piperazines e.g. chlorcyclizine.
5. Phenothiazines e.g. promethazine.

Bradykinin

The most immediate response to tissue injury is probably vasodilatation due to the release of substance P and histamine. Neutrophils migrate along a chemotactic gradient into tissue fluid producing a plasmin activator with the formation of bradykinin. Kinins, including the peptide bradykinin, are highly active in a number of different organs. Bradykinin is thought to play an important role in several pathophysiological conditions including inflammation, pain and shock. It acts not as a blood-borne hormone, but as a local agent, released at or near the site of action by the effect of enzymes (kallikreins) on protein precursors (kininogens). The algesic effect of the kinins is thought to involve direct stimulation of free afferent nerve endings.[18] Bradykinin activates phospholipase A_2 on cell membranes releasing arachidonic acid with the production of a number of prostaglandins.[19] The lipoxygenase products, leukotrienes D_4 and C_4 are also formed. These produce an increase in capillary permeability and further neutrophil activity with the release of more bradykinin.[20] The ability of bradykinin to produce a pain response may be accentuated by prostaglandins which sensitize tissue to the algesic action of bradykinin.

The search for clinically applicable kinin receptor antagonists has been singularly unproductive. The best candidate for therapeutic use has been the polypeptide inhibitor of kallikrein, aprotinin, but this has only been of value in conditions involving excess kinin formation.[21] Peptide analogues of bradykinin have been synthesized and shown to have receptor antagonist properties in appropriate *in vitro* models.[22] Some of these agents notably [Thi[5, 8], D-Phe[7]]-BK, which block the BK_2 receptor for bradykinin will prevent the excitation of polymodal nociceptors by exogenously applied bradykinin although they have not been shown to block the excitation of nociceptors by heat or high K^+ concentrations.[23] Recently it has been shown that BK receptors are induced in inflamed tissues and that a novel antagonist active at both BK_1 and BK_2 receptors (D-Arg[Hyp[3], DPhe[7]]BK) inhibited neurogenic inflammation produced by capsaicin[24]. Whether or not bradykinin receptor antagonists will ever be useful as clinical analgesics can only be determined when stable (probably non-peptide) drugs are available for clinical evaluation.

Serotonin, 5-hydroxytryptamine (5-HT)

It has been known for several decades that intradermal administration of 5-HT mimics the effects of mechanical or chemical injury in man including vasodilatation, oedema formation and the perception of pain. The ability of 5-HT to induce pain is mimicked in a dose-dependent manner by the selective $5-HT_3$ agonist 2-methyl-5HT, and is blocked by selective $5-HT_3$ antagonists, but not by methysergide (which is an antagonist at $5-HT_1$ and $5-HT_2$ receptors). However, there is some evidence which suggests that 5-HT may be of less importance than bradykinin as a mediator of pain and hyperalgesia in inflammation.[25] It is interesting to note that 50 per cent of the $5HT_3$ receptors in the dorsal horn of the rat spinal cord are associated with capsaicin sensitive C-fibre afferents,[26] and that the $5-HT_3$ receptor antagonist ICS 205-930 will prevent the hyperalgesia associated with paw inflammation in the rat at an intraplantar dose of 3.2ng/Kg.[27]

Of the clinically available 5-HT antagonists, only methysergide has any effect upon $5-HT_1$ receptors, but this is a mixture of agonist and antagonist actions and has no general relevance to pain relief.[28] Recently two compounds with agonist activity at $5-HT_{1A}$ receptors (buspirone and m-chlorophenylpiperazine) have been found to be ineffective in patients with neuropathic pain.[29] $5-HT_1$ agonists, namely ergotamine and the selective $5-HT_{1A}$ agonist sumatriptan, will promote vasoconstriction and reduce plasma extravasation[28] within the cerebral circulation and will relieve the pain of migraine. Ketanserin, a $5-HT_2$ antagonist probably exerts an indirect action upon the pain and hypersensitivity of reflex sympathetic dystrophy by its blockade of $5-HT_2$ receptors on vascular smooth muscle. This will promote the restoration of normal peripheral circulatory balance and tissue oxygenation reducing nociceptor stimulation from potassium ions and chemoceptors.[30]

Prostaglandins

Inflammatory pain probably results from the synergistic action of two types of stimulation of the pain receptors, indirect potentiation and direct algesic stimulation. The potentiating stimulus lowers the threshold to mechanical, thermal or chemical stimulation and is probably associated with increased levels of cyclic AMP/Ca^{2+} at the nociceptors.[31] Prostacyclin is probably the most important hyperalgesic mediator present at the site of the inflammatory and tissue damage reaction and other arachidonic acid metabolites contribute to a varying degree.

The nonsteroidal anti-inflammatory drugs (NSAID) inhibit the synthesis of prostaglandins (Fig. 3.1.), and hence the production of hyperalgesia. Aspirin and most of the other NSAID inhibit irreversibly the enzyme, cyclo-oxygenase, by acetylation of a serine residue at the active site of the enzyme. In contrast, the non-acetylated salicyates, e.g. diflunisal trisilate, are almost inactive against cyclo-oxygenase *in vitro*, but are as active as aspirin *in vivo*.[32] For indomethacin, the mode of inhibition is particularly complex and probably involves a site on the enzyme different from that which is acetylated by aspirin. Paracetamol has only weak cyclo-oxygenase inhibitory properties, but has a well marked and used analgesic effect. Clinically, the analgesic potency of the NSAID does not equate with the degree of cyclo-oxygenase inhibition (Table 3.3.). It would appear that the effect upon prostaglandin synthesis is more complex than initially postulated or that the anti-inflammatory and analgesic effects are produced in part by different and separate mechanisms, the latter

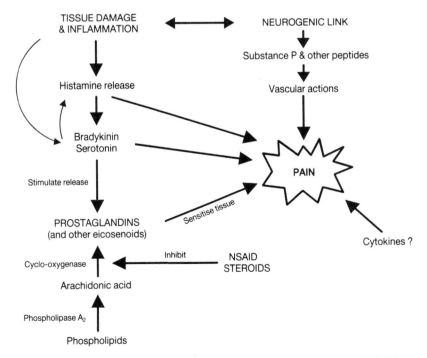

Figure 3.1 Pain production and the role of various mediators and inhibitors.

Table 3.3 Comparison of degree of analgesia exerted by NSAID's with their cyclo-oxygenase inhibition

NSAID in descending analgesic order	Cyclo-oxygenase inhibition umol/l
Diclofenac	1.6
Piroxicam	2.3
Indomethacin	5.6
Naproxen	5.7
Ibuprofen	39.0
Pheylbutazone	490.0
Acetylsalicylic acid	3300.0

Comparison of degree of analgesia exerted by NSAID's with their cyclo-oxygenase inhibition.

of which has yet to be determined (Fig. 3.1.)[33] When defining drug usage to combat pain and inflammation, it still remains a matter of experience rather than applied science as to which NSAID should be prescribed for any particular situation. One of the great advantages of this group of drugs is the variety of formulations available so that application may be by the systemic route – oral, parenteral, rectal or by the topical route.[34, 35] The side effects of NSAID are mainly as a consequence of their pharmocological action affecting the gastro-intestinal system, or more rarely the skin, respiratory, renal and haemopoetic systems. The most important action is probably damage to the gastric mucosa caused by removal of cytoprotective prostaglandins. It is possible that blockade of cyclo-oxygenase shunts arachidonic metabolism into the lipoxygenase pathway leading to enhanced leukotriene production and that this contributes to gastric mucosa damage and causes bronchoconstriction (aspirin asthma).

It should be noted that some recently introduced drugs (e.g. ketorolac) have a higher analgesic efficacy than their ability to inhibit cyclo-oxygenase *in vitro* would suggest to be appropriate, and such drugs may have considerable therapeutic utility.

Substance P

It has been noted previously that the peripheral 'flare and weal' response has been attributed to the release of substance P (SP) and other peptides (notably calcitonin gene related peptide) from peripheral sensory fibres in turn acting on mast cells to release histamine. In addition, sensory nerve endings are sensitized to the action of locally released algesic substances. SP also may contribute to the severity of joint inflammation as the concentration of SP increases in branches of peripheral nerves innervating inflamed joints.[36] SP has been shown to stimulate, in a dose-dependent manner, the release of prostaglandin E_2 from synoviocytes obtained from rheumatoid arthritis patients. Thus, the local release of SP may contribute to the tissue destruction and pain associated with arthritis.[10] Recently, it has been shown that direct intraplantar injection of nanogram doses of SP produces a long lasting hyperalgesia in the rat paw. Interestingly, it was shown that this action or the similar hyperalgesia produced by intraplantar injection of the eicosanoids PGE_2 and prostacyclin could be equally well prevented by pretreatment with the SP receptor antagonist (D-Arg[1], DPro[2], DTrp[7, 9] Leu[11])-SP. This suggests not only that SP might have a role as a modulator in peripheral inflammatory pain but that some of the actions of eicosanoids might be exerted indirectly through SP.[37]

Capsaicin, the pungent constituent of red peppers, is well known to cause pain when applied to the tissues in animals and in man (see reference 38 for a recent review). This action is present in normal individuals and in elderly patients with chronic pain and is believed to be due to a selective C-fibre afferent stimulation leading to release of SP and other peptides within the dorsal horn of the spinal cord.[39] Recently a very potent capsaicin-like nociceptor stimulator called resiniferatoxin has been described and this will undoubtedly assist elucidation of structure–activity relationships for agents of this type.[40] The stimulant action of capsaicin and analogues such as resiniferatoxin is followed by a prolonged period of desensitization when the nociceptor is insensitive to further application of capsaicin or to noxious stimuli.[38, 40] Clinical studies using topical capsaicin in patients with de-afferentation pain have been promising. The selective nature of the action of the agent in reducing just C-nociceptor activity may make it particularly useful for treating pain states triggered by C-fibre input.[38] Analogues of capsaicin are now becoming available that are antinociceptive without causing an initial nociceptor stimulation and such agents have considerable therapeutic potential.[41]

Opioids

Whilst in the normal situation the antinociceptive activity of exogenous opioids is generally agreed to be mediated centrally, in rats with artificially induced inflamed paws at least a component of the analgesic action of opioids appears to be mediated by activation of receptors within the inflamed peripheral tissue.[42] In similar animals, stress-induced antinociception was found to be naloxone reversible with a significantly higher degree of analgesia seen in the inflamed paw when compared with the normal. This differential analgesia is mediated, at least in part, by activation of peripheral opioid receptors by endogenous ligands, the activity of which is dependent upon the integrity of the hypophysis but not that of the adrenal glands. This finding has yet to be followed up clinically in man but with the emergence of the use of topically applied opioids in clinical practice, their use in arthritic patients may now be logical.[43]

Axonal malfunction

Pain due to axonal malfunction may have a number of different aetiologies:

1.　Total or partial severance of the nerve by trauma, surgery or avulsion.
2.　Compression or distortion by oedema, tumour or scar tissue.
3.　Metabolic, chemical or neoplastic neuropathy.
4.　Axonal damage following infection, e.g. post herpetic neuralgia.
5.　Ideopathic malfunction, e.g. trigeminal neuralgia.

This wide spectrum of causative factors and the differing types of lesions produced necessitates the use of therapeutic agents with a variety of actions in order to attempt to cope with the pain (see Table 3.4).[44]

Table 3.4　Therapeutic agents

Steroids	Dexamethasone, betamethasone
Anticonvulsants	Carbamazepine, sodium valproate, baclofen, clonazepam
Tricycle antidepressants	Amitriptyline, nortriptyline
Phenothiazine derivatives	Perphenazine, pericyazine
Serotonin antagonists	Ketanserin
Adrenergic antagonists	Propranolol, labetolol
Adrenergic neurone blockers	Guanethidine, bretylium
Amide local anaesthetic analogues	Tocainide, flecainide
Calcium channel blockers	Nifedipine, diltiazem
Enzyme inhibitors	Aldose reductase inhibitors.

Steroids

Steroids are of value whenever a nerve is subjected to irritation from a solid body in a confined space. This may be a nerve root moving over an osteophyte in the intervertebral foramen or when compressed between a tumour and a solid structure such as bone. Pressure or irritation of the nerve will produce oedema which in itself will increase the pressure on the nervous tissue and hence generate or increase pain.[45] Spinal neoplastic secondaries may produce similar pressure effects on axons, not only by their bulk but also by possible bony infiltration causing collapse of a vertebral body with subsequent pressure on a nerve root. Steroids will act to decrease the oedema of both the nerve and the bulk of the tumour. Dexamethasone or betamethasone are the agents most often used in such situations, given either intravenously or by mouth. Improvement both in pain and neurological status may be seen in as short a time as 12 hours.

Anticonvulsants

These agents used in the treatment of peripheral axonal malfunction are most readily subdivided by their chemical classification (Table 3.5). Whilst all of these agents are loosely categorized as anticonvulsants, the actual site and mode of action vary such that their usage and indications for clinical use are not identical.[46] Carbamazepine and phenytoin are used extensively for the treatment of the cranial nerve neuralgias and some of the peripheral neuropathies. They both bind to specific 'phenytoin-recognizing-receptors' producing voltage-sensitive sodium channel inactivation and an opening of chloride channels thereby stabilizing the cell near its resting membrane potential.[44, 47, 48, 49, 50, 51, 52] The only two benzodiazepines with proven analgesic activity, clonazepam and clobazam, bind with a dedicated site on the GABA-A receptor complex facilitating GABA-mediated transmission.[53] Clonazepam is valuable in treating facial and post-traumatic neurogenic pain whilst clobazam is mainly used for peripheral neuropathies and de-afferentation. Sodium valproate is used again in traumatic and other neuropathies and is thought to work, at least in part, by augmenting GABA-mediated inhibitory transmission.[54, 55]

Table 3.5   Anticonvulsants

Hydantoins	Phenytoin sodium.
Benzodiazepines	Clonazepam, clobazam.
Iminostilbines	Carbamazepine.
Carboxylic acids	Sodium valproate

Tricyclic antidepressants

The tricyclic antidepressants have a wide range of actions affecting many neurotransmitters both centrally and in the periphery. At one extreme the effects of serotonin may be enhanced by blocking the presynaptic re-uptake, whilst at the other, a marked anticholinergic action is seen from the more analgesic members of the group. The use of such agents is well documented in the literature and whilst their use has been ubiquitous the defined indications for use are less clear.[56, 59] Suffice it to say that in cases of peripheral neuropathy from whatever cause, tricyclics in combination with either anticonvulsants or phenothiazine derivatives are a first line choice.

The dose range over which they exert their effect is wide and because of the sometimes problematic side effects, especially in the old and frail, the optimal dose should be built up to slowly. Use can be made of the hypnotic effect and when initiating medication, the agent of choice may be given only at night for the first week or two of treatment. As there are many tricyclics available it should be emphasized that the older agents with a width of neurotransmitter activity are more active and of greater clinical value than the transmitter specific, newer agents.[33]

Phenothiazine derivatives

The phenothiazine derivatives are mainly used in combination with either tricyclic antidepressant agents in the treatment of peripheral neuropathies or with opioid agents to enhance their analgesic activity and reduce certain of the side effects. The phenothiazines have certain similarities to the tricyclics in that the older agents with a wider spectrum of interaction with different neurotransmitter receptors have proved to be the best clinically. This has been suggested as being due to their dopamine antagonism, anticholinergic effect, antihistaminergic activity or their local anaesthetic-like effect upon peripheral nerves. It is most likely to be a combination of all of these with an optimal degree of effect on each system.[60, 62] Because the phenothiazines are so often used in combination with the antidepressants, the same constraints on their clinical usage apply.

Serotonin antagonists

To date, the most effective agent for use in de-afferentation pain has been ketanserin. This has an antagonist effect at peripheral $5\text{-}HT_2$ receptors, apparently restoring the normal function of the microcirculation, disrupted by vasoconstriction which is $5\text{-}HT_2$ receptor mediated. 5-HT can also facilitate or amplify the vasoconstrictor effect of other agents such as angiotensin II or catecholamines. This effect is also $5\text{-}HT_2$ receptor mediated and can be blocked by ketanserin. The malfunction of the microcirculation leads to persistent dilatation of the arterio-venous shunts such that tissue hypoxia results. The fall in pH, enhanced by the loss of acid-base buffer enables hydrogen ions to bind to haemoglobin in the red cells with the release of potassium ions which may activate nociceptors producing pain. 5-HT will also produce an increase in transmitter release from sensory fibre terminals, an action that is also blocked by ketanserin.[20, 63, 65] Ketanserin also has a significant α_1 adrenoceptor blocking effect and this will contribute to the restoration of normal circulatory function both in peripheral tissue and in the vicinity of sensory axons.[64]

Other 5-HT receptor blockers such as methysergide and mianserin have no effect upon deafferentation problems, possibly due to a lesser anti-adrenergic effect or the lack of investigation due to the absence of a parenteral formulation.[65, 66]

Adrenergic antagonists

Damage to an axon can produce ectopic foci of discharges anywhere along its length.[67] In addition, areas of demyelination or abnormal myelin may develop ephaptic foci with crosstalk between adjacent fibres and continuous discharges. The relative preponderance of C fibres biases the response of axonal damage towards the development of pain. Damage to large diameter fibres may result in a loss of their inhibitory activity on C-fibre excitation of spinal dorsal horn neurones. The damaged axon not only shows abnormal impulse generation but is also abnormally sensitive to noradrenaline which may well be the pathological basis for hyperpathia.[68]

The effectiveness of propranolol in the treatment of certain peripheral nerve disorders such as phantom limb pain, post-traumatic pain and post herpetic neuralgia has been described.[69, 70, 71] In common with the situation in migraine, not all beta adrenergic antagonists have a beneficial effect.[43] Those without intrinsic sympathomimetic activity would appear to be preferred together with a degree of mixed alpha and beta effect. It may be the ratio of the alpha and beta blocking effects that are of vital importance to the peripheral analgesic activity. Labetalol as well as propranolol falls into this category and it is of interest that abrupt withdrawal of these agents may induce clinical symptoms suggesting adrenergic hypersensitivity.[72] This peripheral effect may be enhanced by a central action involving beta receptors. It should also be noted that a number of the agents mentioned above can block Ca^{2+} channels and this too could contribute to their therapeutic action in the analgesic context.

Adrenergic neurone blockers

An important factor in nerve injury pain is the influence of the sympathetic nervous system. Patients with chronic pain of this origin may be divided into two categories; those with sympathetically maintained pain (SMP) and those whose pain is independent of sympathetic activity (SIP). The diagnosis of SMP is made when the pain and hyperalgesia is removed by blockade of the sympathetic efferents.[73] Sympathetic efferent activity which normally evokes ongoing firing in low-threshold mechanoceptors, following injury will evoke a response in wide dynamic range neurones in the dorsal horn which, due to the injury, have an enhanced responsiveness to low-threshold mechanoceptor activity. Sympathetic efferent activity may also directly activate nociceptors to account for the ongoing pain in SMP. The pain in SMP may, therefore, be significantly relieved by drugs interfering with alpha-adrenergic function. These include guanethidine,[74] bretyllium,[75] reserpine,[76] phenoxybenzamine,[77] and prazosin.[78] The usual mode of administration of these agents is by the isolated limb perfusion technique.[74] The mode of action appears to be that guanethidine accumulates in and displaces noradrenaline from intraneuronal storage granules.[78] Reserpine reduces the re-uptake of catecholamines whilst being itself accumulated in intraterminal storage granules. Bretylium exerts multiple effects on the metabolism of noradrenaline and blocks its release following nerve stimulation in addition to being a potent inhibitor of uptake into terminals.

Amide local anaesthetic analogues

The value of intravenous lignocaine for treating chronic pain has been well documented for a number of years.[79] The mechanism of action has been variously suggested as an antagonistic action to neurotransmitters,[80] a reduction in neuronal depolarization or a decrease in high frequency transmission.[81, 82] For chronic use, however, the intravenous route of administration poses a number of problems. The introduction of orally administered analogues of the amide local anaesthetics, mexiletine, tocainide and flecainide has, to a great extent, solved the problem. Their use in the treatment of neuralgias and peripheral neuropathies has been shown to be a useful addition to the analgesic armamentarium.[83–85]

Calcium channel blockers

It has been shown in several experimental models that both the mu and kappa opioid receptor agonists interact indirectly with the presynaptic terminal calcium channel and modulate neurotransmitter release. Whilst the mu agonist effect is indirect by increasing potassium efflux, that of the kappa agonist directly decreases the calcium influx.[86, 87] As the above analgesic agents could (by some stretch of the imagination!) be considered to act as calcium channel blockers, it was suggested that classical calcium channel blockers might act as analgesic agents. This has subsequently been shown to be so and both nifedipine and diltiazem are used for the treatment of SMP, Raynaud's disease and peripheral neuropathies.[88–90]

Enzyme inhibitors

Disabling pain is one of the serious consequences of diabetic neuropathy. The whole condition is characterized by a distal, symmetrical, mixed sensorimotor type of neural deficit with decrease of both motor and sensory nerve conduction. The primary deficit is due to non-optimal glycemic control leading to an excessive accumulation of sorbitol and other polyols within Schwann cells, axons and perineural space.[91] Aldose reductase, the rate-limiting enzyme of the polyol pathway, found only in Schwann cells, catalyses the formation of alcohol sugars from hexose sugars or aldoses. The substrate affinity of the enzyme is so low that substantial intracellular accumulation of sorbitol occurs only when intracellular levels of glucose are high. This alcohol sugar does not permeate the cell membrane and persists for long periods probably causing, at least in part, the neuropathology.[92] Agents which inhibit aldose reductase have been shown to increase the affected nerve conduction velocities in diabetics together with a significant and lasting reduction in sensory and motor impairment.[91, 92, 93, 94]

Dorsal root ganglion

The dorsal root ganglion (DRG) is the location of the cell bodies for the afferent peripheral sensory nerves. The majority of these, some 70 per cent, will pursue their expected course in the posterior spinal root and enter the dorsal horn of the cord to synapse in the substantia gelatinosa and deeper laminae. The remaining 30 per cent will, perhaps unexpectedly, pass from the DRG and enter the cord via the anterior spinal root eventually reaching the same terminus as their fellows.[95] Temporary or permanent lesions of the DRG will block the afferent sensory pathway completely. This is not seen when surgical rhizotomy is performed proximal to the DRG as only the 70 per cent of afferents passing in the posterior root will be sectioned.[96] The DRG is, therefore, the most suitable site for lesioning the peripheral sensory pathway and especially so for permanent denervation because the destruction of the cell bodies within the DRG will prevent regrowth of nervous tissue and the possibility of restoration of function. Temporary changes of function of the DRG may be produced by the injection of local anaesthetic solution around the DRG.[97] Irritation of the nerve root in the inter-vertebral foramen with the resultant oedema may be caused by osteophytes or tumor. Instillation of a suitable steroid around the DRG frequently reduces this oedema, allows normal nerve function to take place and reduces or obtunds the pain. The steroids most often used are methylprednisolone, triamcinolone or dexamethasone.[98, 99] Irreversible lesions of the DRG may be produced mechanically, by the use of radio-frequency thermocoagulation or by cryotherapy.[100, 101] Alternative destructive lesions may be induced by the use of neurolytic chemicals injected around the DRG in a manner similar to that described in reference 97. The agent most commonly used is phenol, either in a 5–7 per cent solution in glycerine or, less frequently, in aqueous solution. Small volumes only should be used to minimize the risk of spread on to adjacent structures and care must be taken to ensure that the injectate is deposited epidurally. Glycerine alone can also be injected around the DRG to produce a slow developing lesion. A volume of up to 0.5 ml anhydrous glycerine is used and the benefit may take up to 72 hours to develop. In common with other neurolytic therapy, post lesion neuritis may develop but will gradually diminish over the course of several weeks.[97]

Dorsal horn of the spinal cord

Many centrally acting analgesics, notably the opioids, exert part of their action within the dorsal horn of the spinal cord either to reduce the amount of transmitter release from nociceptor fibre terminals or to directly reduce the excitability of the relay neurones within the spinal cord.[102] There is evidence that both μ and δ opioid agonists can produce analgesia in man by an action at the spinal level[103] but at present it is an open question as to whether κ agonists will work at this site as there is some controversy in the literature over spinal κ antinociception in animals that is likely to be explicable in terms of interspecies and developmental differences.[102, 104] Drugs that share a common mechanism of intracellular action with the opioids, although they do not bind to opioid receptors, can be shown to produce analgesia by an action, at least in part, within the dorsal horn of the spinal cord. The best known drugs of this type are clonidine and baclofen which have the ability to increase outward K^+ conductance in spinal dorsal horn neurones in a similar manner to μ opioids (see for example reference 105). The therapeutic utility of such agents seems to be limited by unwanted side effects such as depression of blood pressure that are evident at the analgesic dose and this is probably related to a more widespread anatomical location of α_2 and $GABA_B$ receptors than of opioid receptors.

There has been considerable interest recently in the possibility that the peptide cholecystokinin (CCK) might have an endogenous anti-opioid role within the spinal dorsal horn and there is also some evidence that CCK might, paradoxically, also have analgesic properties of its own.[106] This latter hypothesis is given support by the observation that CCK can release the inhibitory transmitter GABA within the spinal cord[107] but it is more therapeutically relevant to note that the potent CCK-B receptor antagonist L-365260 will enhance morphine analgesia and prevent the development of morphine tolerance in the rat and may thus be a lead toward novel analgesic medication.[108]

Much of the impulse traffic into the dorsal horn is carried by way of excitatory amino acid neurotransmitters and it has been shown that antagonists of excitatory amino acid receptors can produce antinociception in animals[109] and that this effect may be modality selective.[110] The ubiquitous nature of excitatory amino acid operated neurotransmission will probably curtail the therapeutic utility of such agents, however.

Future trends

The range and diversity of chemical messengers that can be associated with nociception continues to increase. For example, it is now known that nerve growth factor as well as being essential for the normal development of sensory neurones can regulate the duration of the action potential in mature sensory neurones, and it has been suggested that this could be important in controlling the response to nerve injury.[111] Indeed, a new neuronal growth factor has been isolated from injured peripheral nerve that both enhances neurite outgrowth and increases myelination.[112]

Molecular biology is starting to make an impact in the pain research field and it is likely that the chronic changes seen on nerve injury or in response to prolonged inflammation are related to gene induction. For example, following 3 weeks of arthritic inflammation in the rat there is an increase in levels of mRNA coding for the production of pro-opiomelanocortin, the precursor of β-endorphin,[113] and pro-dynorphin gene expression in rat spinal cord is enhanced after traumatic injury.[114] Shorter time course events including acute noxious stimuli, will cause induction of the c-fos proto-oncogene.[115] It has been determined that c-fos mRNA levels rise in rat spinal cord immediately on production of inflammation in a paw[116] and that analgesic drugs such as morphine may be able to suppress such c-fos induction.[117] The clinical relevance of such observations may not be immediately obvious but this is an extremely fast-moving area of research and the increase in the number of possible sites for therapeutic intervention will almost certain lead to new treatment strategies within the next decade.

References

1. White J. C., Sweet W. H. *Pain and the neurosurgeon* Springfield, Illinois: Thomas, 1969.
2. Lynn B. The detection of injury and tissue damage. In: Wall P. D., Melzack R. (eds) *Pain* London: Churchill Livingstone, 1984.
3. Burgess P. R., Perl E. R. Myelinated afferent fibres responding specifically to noxious stimulation of the skin *J. Physiol.* 1967; **190**: 541–62.
4. Bessou P., Perl E. R. Response of cutaneous sensory units with unmyelinated fibres to noxious stimuli *J. Neurophysiol.* 1969; **32**: 1025–43.
5. Chahl L. A. *Mechanisms of Pain and Analgesic Compounds.* Burs, Bennet, (eds) New York: Raven Press, 1979.
6. Hokfeldt T., Vincent S. Dalsgaard, C-J., Skirbou L., Johansson, O. Schultzberg, M. Lunberg, J. M., Roseu, S. Janeso, G. Distribution of substance P in brain and periphery and its possible role as co-transmitter. In: *Substance P in the Nervous System.* Porter, O'Conner (eds) Ciba Symposium 91. London: Pitman, 1982: 84–100.
7. Lynn B. Cutaneous hyperalgesia. *Brit Med. Bull.* 1977; **33**: 103–8.

8. Lembeck F., Donnerer J. Post occlusive cutaneous vasodilation mediated via Substance P. *Naunyn Schmeidebergs Arch. Pharmacol.* 1981; **316**: 165–71.
9. Ryall R. W. *Mechanism of Drug Action in the Nervous System*, 2nd ed. Cambridge: Cambridge University Press, 1989.
10. Raja S. N., Mayer R. A., Campbell J. N. Peripheral mechanisms of somatic pain. *Anesthesiology.* 1988; **68**: 571–90.
11. Moncada S. Biological importance of prostacyclin. *Brit. J. Pharmacol.* 1982; **76**: 3–31.
12. Juan H. Mechanism of action of bradykinin-induced release of prostaglandin E. *Naunyn Schmeidebergs Arch. Pharmacol.* 1977; **300**: 77–85.
13. White, D. M., Basbaum, A. I., Goetzl, E. J., Levine, J. D. 8(R), 15(S) - diHETE sensitizes C-fibre nociceptors in the hairy skin of the rat. *Soc Neurosci Abs.* 1989; 15 471.
14. Follenfant, R. L. Nakamura-Craig, M. Henderson, B. Higgs G. A. Inhibition by neuropeptides of interleukin – 1β-induced prostaglandin-independent hyperalgesia *Br. J. Pharmacol.* 1989; **98**: 41–43.
15. McMahon S. B., Kiltzenburg M. Novel classes of nociceptors; beyond Sherrington. *Trends in Neurosciences.* 1990; **13**: 199–201
16. Douglas W. W. Autacoids. In: *The Pharmacological Basis of Therapeutics.* 6th ed. Eds; Gilman G. G., Goodman L. S., Gilman A. New York. Macmillan; 1980.
17. Casy A. F. Chemistry of anti H_1 histamine antagonists. In: *Histamine 2 and Antihistamines.* Ed; Rocha e Silva M. Handbuch der Experimentahlen Pharmakologie. 1978; **18**: 93–108.
18. Moody T. W., Perry D. C. Peptide receptors. In: *Receptor Pharmacology and Function,* Eds; Williams M, Glennon R. A., Timmermanns P. B. M. New York. Marcel Dekker, 1989; pp 527–570.
19. Singer M. A., Peach M. J. Endothelium-dependent relaxation of rabbit aorta. 1. Relaxation stimulated by arachidonic acid. *J. Pharmacol Exp. Ther.* 1983; **226**: 790–801.
20. Cooke E. D., Ward C. Vicious circles in reflex sympathetic dystrophy–a hypothesis; discussion paper. *J. Roy. Soc. Med.* 1990; **83**: 96–99.
21. Haberland G. L. The role of kininogenases, kinin formation and kininogenase inhibition in post traumatic shock and related conditions. *Klin. Wochenschr.* 1978; **56**: 325–331.
22. Vavrek R. J., Stewart J. M. Competitive antagonists of bradykinin. *Peptides* 1985; **6**: 161–4.
23. Mizumura K., Mina Gaira M., Tsuji'i T., Kumazaira J. The effects of bradykinin agonists and antagonists on visceral polymodal receptor activities *Pain* 1990; **40**: 221–7.
24. Mantione C. R., Rodriguez R. A bradykinin (BK_1) receptor antagonist blocks capsaicin-induced ear inflammation in mice. *Br. J. Pharmacol* 1990; **99**: 516–8.
25. Beck P. W., Handwerker, H. O. Bradykinin and serotonin effects on various types of cutaneous nerve fibre. *Pflugers Arch.* 1974; **347**: 209–22.
26. Hamon M., Gallisot M. E., Menard F., Gozlan K., Bourgoin S., Verge D. 5-HT_3 receptor binding sites are on capsaicin-sensitive fibres in the rat spinal cord. *Eur. J. Pharmacol.* 1989; **164**: 315–22.
27. Eschalier A., Kayser V., Guilbaud G. Influence of a specific 5-HT_3-antagonist on carrageen-induced hyperalgesia in rats. *Pain* 1989; **36**:

249–55.

28. Buzzi M G. Moskowitz M. A. The antimigraine drug, sumatriptan (GR43175), selectively blocks neurogenic plasma extravasation from blood vessels in dura mater. *Br. J. Pharmacol.* 1990; **99**: 202–6.

29. Kishore-Kumar R., Schafter S. C., Lawlor B. A., Murphy, D. L., Niar B. B. Single doses of the serotonin agonists buspirone and m-chloro-phenylpiperazine do not relieve neuropathic pain. *Pain* 1989; **37**: 223–7.

30. Peatfield R. C. Drugs in the treatment of migraine. *Trends in Pharm. Sci.* 1988; **9**: 141–5.

31. Ferreira S. H., Nakamura M. Prostaglandin hyperalgesia. A cAMP/Ca²⁺ dependent process. *Prostaglandins* 1979; **18**: 179–90.

32. Hamberg M. Inhibition of prostaglandin synthesis in man *Biochem. Biophys. Res. Comm.* 1972; **49**: 720–6.

33. Budd K. The pain clinic-chronic pain. In: *General Anaesthesia*, 5th ed. Eds: Nunn J. F., Utting J. E., Brown B. R., London, Butterworth.

34. King R. B. Concerning the management of pain associated with herpes zoster and of post herpetic neuralgia. *Pain* 1988; **39**: 73–8.

35. Kassirer M. R. Concerning the management of pain associated with herpes zoster and post herpetic neuralgia. *Pain* 1988; **35**: 368–9.

36. Lembeck F., Donner J. Increase of SP in primary afferent nerve during chronic pain. *Neurophysiol.* 1981; **1**: 175–80.

37. Nakamura-Craig M., Smith T. W., Substance P and peripheral inflammatory hyperalgesia. *Pain* 1989; **38**: 91–8.

38. Lynn B. Capsaicin: actions on nociceptive C fibres and therapeutic potential. *Pain* 1990; **41**: 61–9.

39. Levasseur S. A., Gibson S. J., Neline R. D. The measurement of capsaicin-sensitive nerve fibre function in elderly patients with pain. *Pain* 1990; **41**: 19–25.

40. Dray A., Bettaney J., Foster D. Resiniferatoxin, a potent capsaicin-like stimulator of peripheral nociceptors in the neonatal rat tail *'in vitro' Br. J. Pharmacol.* 1990; **99**: 323–6.

41. Dray A., Bettaney J., Rueff A., Walpole C., and Ungglearonn, K. NE-19550 and NE-21610, antinociceptive capsaicin analogues: studies on nociceptive fibres of the neonatal rat tail *'in vitro' Eur. J. Pharmacol* 1990; **181**: 289–93.

42. Parsons C. G., Celonikowski A., Stein C., Herz A. Peripheral opioid receptors mediating antinociception in inflammation *Pain*. 1990; **41**: 81–93.

43. Nimmo W. S. The promise of transdermal drug delivery. *Brit. J. Anaesth.* 1990; **64**: 7–10.

44. Casey K. L. Towards a rationale for the treatment of painful neuropathies. In: *Proceedings of the 5th World Congress on Pain.* Eds: Dubner R., Gebhart G. F., Bond M. R. 1988; 165–74. Amsterdam, Elsevier.

45. Twycross R. G., LACK S. *Symptom Control in Far Advanced Cancer: Pain Relief.* 1983; 270–93. London, Pitman.

46. Budd K. Sodium valproate in the treatment of pain. In: *4th International Congress on Sodium Valproate and Epilepsy.* Ed: Chadwick D. 1989; 213–6. Royal Society of Medicine International Congress & Symposium Series 152, London, R. Soc. Med.

47. Bada J. L., Cervera C., Padro L. Carbamazepine for amyloid neuropathy. *New England J. Med.* 1977; **296**: 396.

48. Portnoy R. K. Duma C., Foley K. M. Acute herpetic and post herpetic neuralgia clinical review and current management. *Ann. Neurol.* 1986; **20**: 651–64.

49. Fromm G. H., Terrence C. F., Maroon J. C. Trigeminal neuralgia; current concepts regarding etiology and pathogenesis. *Arch. Neurol.* 1984; **41**: 1204–7.

50. Maclean M. J., MacDonald R. L. Multiple actions of phenytoin in mouse cord neurones in cell culture. *J. Pharmacol. and Exp. Ther.* 1983; **227**: 779–89.

51. Ibid. Carbamazepine and 10, 11, epoxycarbamazepine produce use and voltage-dependent limitation of rapidly firing action potentials of mouse central neurones in cell culture. *J. Pharmacol. Exp. Ther.* 1986; **238**: 727–38.

52. Willow M. Pharmacology of diphenylhydantoin and carbamazepine action on voltage sensitive sodium channels. *Trends in Neurosc.* 1986; **9**: 147–9.

53. Suria A., Costa E. Evidence for GABA involvement in the action of diazepam on presynaptic nerve terminals in bullfrog sympathetic ganaglia. *Adv. Biochem. Psychopharmacol.* 1975; **14**: 103–12.

54. Swerdlow M., Cundill J. G. Anticonvulsant drugs used in the treatment of lancinating pain. A comparison. *Anaesthesia* 1981; **36**: 1129-32.

55. MacDonald R. L., Bergey G. K. Valproic acid augments GABA-mediated post-synaptic inhibition in cultured mammalian neurones. *Brain Res.* 1979; **170**: 558–62.

56. Monks R., Merskey H. Psychotropic drugs, in: *Textbook of Pain* Eds: Wall P., Melzack R. 1984; 526–37. Edinburgh, Churchill-Livingstone.

57. Feinmann C. Pain relief by antidepressants: possible modes of action. *Pain.* 1985; **23**: 1–8.

58. Taub A., Collins W. F. Observations on the treatment of denervation dysaethesia with psychotropic drugs. In: *Advances in Neurology*, Vol 4. Ed: Bonica J. J. 1974; 309–15. New York. Raven Press.

59. Max M. B., Cykbabem N., Schafer, S. C., Gracely K. H., Waltner D. S. Smailer B., Dubner K. Amitriptyline relieves diabetic neuropathy pain in patients with normal or depressed mood. *Neurol.* 1987; **37**: 589–96.

60. Pert A. Cholinergic and catecholaminergic mechanisms in pain. In: *Neurotransmitters and Pain Control.* Eds: Akil H., Lewis J. W. 1987; 1–6 Basel, Karger.

61. Lasagna R. G., DeKornfield T. J. Methotrimeprazine: A new phenothiazine derivative with analgesic properties. *Jnl. Amer. Med. Assoc.* 1961; **178**: 887–90.

62. Nathan P. W. Chlorprothixene (Taractan) in post-herpetic neuralgia and other severe chronic pains. *Pain* 1978; **5**: 367–71.

63. Timmermanns P. B. M. W. M. Alpha-adrenoceptors. In: *Receptor Pharmacology and Function.* Eds: Williams M., Glennon R. A., Timmermans P. B M. W. M. 1989; 173–205. New York, Dekker.

64. Roberts M. H. T. Pharmacology of putative neurotransmitters and receptors: 5HT. In: *Progress in Brain Research.* Eds: Field H. L., Besson J. M., 1988; 329–338. Amsterdam, Elsevier.

65. Hanna M., Peat S. J. Ketanserin in reflex sympathetic dystrophy. A double-blind, placebo-controlled crossover trial. *Pain* 1989; **38**: 145–50.

66. De Cree J., Leempoels J., Genkens H., Verhaegen K. Placebo-controlled

double blind trial of ketanserin in treatment of intermittent claudication. *Lancet*. 1984; **ii**: 775–8.

67. Ochoa J. L., Torebjork H. E. Paraesthesiae from ectopic impulses generated in human sensory nerves. *Brain* 1986; **103**: 835–53.

68. Wynn-Parry C. B., Withrington R. The management of painful peripheral nerve disorders. In: *Textbook of Pain*. Eds: Wall P. D., Melzack R. 1984; 395–401. Edinburgh, Churchill-Livingstone.

69. Marsland A. R., Weekes J. W. N., Atkinson R. L., Leong, M. G. Phantom limb pain–a case for Blockers. *Pain*. 1982; **12**: 295–7.

70. Scadding J. W., Wall P. D *et al*. Clinical trial of propranolol in post-traumatic neuralgia. *Pain* **14**: 283–92.

71. Visitsunthorn U., Prete P. Reflex sympathetic dystrophy of the lower extremity. A complication of herpes zoster with dramatic response to propranolol *Western Med. J*. 1981; **135**: 62–6.

72. Brodde O. Beta adrenoceptors. In: *Receptor Pharmacology and Function*. Eds: Williams M., Glennon R. A., Timmermanns P. B. M. W. M. 1989; 207–55. New York, Dekker.

73. Campbell J. N., Raja S. N., Meyer R. A. Painful sequelae of nerve injury. In: *Proceedings of the 5th World Congress on Pain*. Eds: Dubner R, Gerbhart G. F, Bond M. R. 1988; 135–43. Amsterdam, Elsevier.

74. Hannington-Kiff J. G. Intravenous regional sympathetic block with guanethidine. *Lancet*. 1974; i; 1019–20

75. Hannington-Kiff J. G. Antisympathetic drugs in limbs. In: *Textbook of Pain*. Eds: Wall P. D., Melzack R., 1984; 566–73.

76. Gorsky B. H. Intravenous perfusion with reserpine for Raynauds phenomenon. *Regional Anesthesia*. 1977; **2**: 5.

77. Ghostine S. Y., Comair Y. G. *et al*. Phenoxybenzamine in the treatment of causalgia. *J. Neurosurg*. 1984; **60**: 1263–8.

78. Benson H. T., Chomka C. M., Brunner E. A. Treatment of reflex sympathetic dystrophy with regional intravenous reserpine. *Anesthesia and Analgesia*. 1980; **59**: 500–1.

79. Swerdlow M. The use of local anesthetics for chronic pain. *The Pain Clinic*. 1988; **2**: 3–6.

80. Edwards W. T., Habib F. *et al*. Intravenous lidocaine in the management of various chronic pain states. *Regional Anesthesia*. 1985; **10**: 1–6.

81. Boas R. A., Corvino B. G., Shahnarian A. Analgesic responses to *i.v.* lignocaine. *Brit. J. Anaesthesia*. 1982; **54**: 501–5.

82. Condouris G. A. Local anesthetics as modulators of neural information. *Adv. Pain Res. Therapy*. 1976; **1**: 663–8.

83. Dejgard A., Petersen P., Kastrup J. Mexiletine for the treatment of chronic painful diabetic neuropathy. *Lancet*. 1988; **i**: 9–11.

84. Dunlop R., Davies R. J., Hockley J., Turner, P. Analgesic effects of oral flecainide. *Lancet*. 1988; **i**: 420–1.

85. Lindstrom P., Lindblom U. The analgesic effect of tocainide in trigeminal neuralgia. *Pain*. 1987; **28**: 45–50.

86. North R. A. Opioid receptor types and membranes on ion channels, *Trends in Neurosci* 1986; **9**: 174–6.

87. Haynes L. Opioid receptors and signal transduction. *Trends in Pharmacol. Sci*. 1988; **9**: 309–11.

88. Hoffmeister F., Tettenborn D. Calcium agonists and antagonists of the dyhydropyidine type. *Psychopharmacol*. 1980; **90**: 299–302.

89. Singhvi I. S., Gershin S. Brain calcium and morphine *Biochem. Pharmacol.* 1977; **20**: 1183–8.

90. Carta F., Bianchi M. *et al.* Effect of nifedipine on morphine induced analgesia. *Anesthesia and Analgesia.* 1990; **70**: 493–8.

91. Handlesman D. J., Turtle J. R. Clinical trial of an aldose reductase inhibitor in diabetic neuropathy. *Diabetes.* 1981; **30**: 459–64,

92. Jaspan J., Marselli R., Kent K., Barthus C. The treatment of severely painful diabetic neuropathy with an aldose reductase inhibitor. *Lancet.* 1983; **ii**: 758–62.

93. Judzewitsch R. G., Jaspan J. *et al.* Aldose reductase inhibition improves nerve conduction velocity in diabetic patients. *New England J. Med.* 1983; **308**: 119–25.

94. Culebras A., Alio J., Kerrera J-L., Lopez-Fraile I. P. Effect of an aldose reductase inhibitor on diabetic peripheral neuropathy *Arch. Neurol.* 1981; **38**: 133–4.

95. Wall P. D. The future of attacks on pain. In: *Pain.* Ed: Bonica J. J. 1974; 301–8. New York, Raven Press.

96. Coggeshall R. E., Applebaum M. B., Fazen M., Stubbs T. B., Sykes M. T. Unmyelinated axons in human ventral roots, a possible explanation for the failure of dorsal rhizotomy to relieve pain. *Brain.* 1975; **98**: 157–66.

97. Budd K. Ablative nerve blocks and neurosurgical techniques. In: *Anaesthesia.* Eds: Nimmo W. S., Smith G. 1989; 1243–66. Blackwell Scientific Publications, Oxford.

98. Kepes E. R., Duncalf D. Treatment of backache with spinal injections of local anesthetics, spinal and systemic steroids. A review. *Pain* 1985; **22**: 33–47.

99. Forest J. B. The response to epidural steroid injections in chronic dorsal root pain. *Canadian Anaesthetists Soc. J.* 1980; **27**: 40–46.

100. Nash T. P. Percutaneous radiofrequency lesioning of dorsal root ganglia for chronic pain. *Pain* 1986; **24**: 67–74.

101. Charlton J. E. Nerve blocking in chronic pain. In *Therapy of Pain.* Ed, Swerdlow M. 1986; 133–64. Lancaster, MTP Press Limited.

102. Hill R. G., Hughes J. Opioid analgesics: CNS sites and mechanisms of action. *Adv. Biosci.* 1989; **75**: 411–4.

103. Hill R. G. New analgesics–a status report. *Curr. Opinion in Anaesth.* 1988; **1**: 367–71.

104. Leighton G. E. *et al.* κ-opioid agonists produce antinociception after *i.v.* and *i.c.v.* but not intrathecal administration in the rat. *Brit. J. Pharmacol.* 1988; **93**: 553–560.

105. Allerton C. A. *et al.* Actions of the GABA$_B$ agonist (-) baclofen, on neurones in deep dorsal horn of the rat spinal cord 'in vitro'. *Brit. J. Pharmacol.* 1989; **96**: 29–38.

106. Pittaway K. M., Hill R. G. Cholecystokinin and pain *Pain Headache* 1987; **9**: 213–46.

107. Rodriguez R. E. *et al.* Cholecystokinin releases (^{3}H) GABA from the perfused subarachnoid space of the anesthetized rat spinal cord. *Neurosci. Lett.* 1987; **83**: 173–8.

108. Dourish C. T. *et al.* The selective CCK-B receptor antagonist L365260 enhances morphine analgesia and prevents morphine tolerance in the rat. *Eur. J. Pharmacol.* 1990; **176**: 35–44.

109. Cahusac P. M. B., Evans R. H., Hill R. G., Rodriguez R. E., Smith

D. A. S. The behavioural effects of an N-Methylaspartate receptor antagonist following application to the lumbar spinal cord of conscious rats. *Neuropharmacol.* 1984; **23**: 719–24.

110. Salt T. E., Hill R. G. Pharmacological differentiation between responses of rat medullary dorsal horn neurones to noxious mechanical and noxious thermal cutaneous stimuli. *Brain Res.* 1983; **263**: 167–71.

111. Chalazonitis A., Patterson E. R., Crain S. M. Nerve growth factor regulates the action potential duration of mature sensory neurons. *Proc. Natl. Acad. Sci. USA.* 1987; **84**: 289–93.

112. Windebank A. J., Blexrud M. D., Biological activity of a new neuronal growth factor from injured peripheral nerve. *Dev. Brain Res.* 1989; **49**: 243–51.

113. Millan J. J., Millan M. H., Czlonkowski A., Hout V., Pilcher C. W., Coijpaert F. C. A model of chronic pain in the rat: response of multiple opioid systems to adjuvant-induced arthritis. *J. Neurosci.* 1986; **6**: 899–906.

114. Przewlocki R., Haarman I., Nikolarakis K., Herz A., Holt V., Prodynorphin gene expression in spinal cord is enhanced after traumatic injury in the rat. *Mol. Brain Res.* 1988; **4**: 37–41.

115. Hunt S. P., Pini A., Evan G. Induction of c-fos-like protein in spinal cord neurons following sensory stimulation. *Nature* 1987; **328**: 632–34.

116. Draisci G., Iadarola M. J. Temporal analysis of increases in c-fos, preprodynorphin and preproenkephalin mRNAs in rat spinal cord. *Mol. Brain Res.* 1989; **6**: 31–37.

117. Presley R. W., Menetrey D., Levine J. D., Basbaum A. I. Systemic morphine suppresses noxious-stimulus-evoked Fos protein-like immunoreactivity in the rat spinal cord. *J. Neurosci.* 1990; **10**: 323–35.

4

The effects of pain and its treatment

N. B. Scott

Introduction

The last few years have seen a considerable increase in our knowledge of the pathophysiology of pain. The benefits of complete analgesia and maintenance of organ function postoperatively are accepted. However the clinical management of pain is largely dictated by concern about the side-effects of the drugs and techniques used to treat it. *This has led to an in-between state whereby most clinicians agree that analgesia is poorly prescribed, but prefer to accept this rather than increase time, effort and resources to improve the situation.*

It is important for the reader to appreciate at the outset that, for major surgery, total pain relief is impossible if only one agent and/or one technique is used. However it may be achieved by combining techniques. The three classes of drugs most readily available and widely used for this are the opioids, local anaesthetics and non-steroidal anti-inflammatory agents (NSAID). These drugs have all been available since the turn of the century but it was only recently that all three were employed together following major abdominal surgery, with considerable effect. This was the first study to document *zero* pain and for a considerable postoperative period (four days).[1]

This chapter first reviews the pathophysiology of both somatic and visceral pain within the global context of nociception, and documents the adverse effects of this on major organ function; secondly, it discusses the side-effects of the three classes of drugs to demonstrate their own potential contribution to post operative morbidity; thirdly, it describes the effects that these drugs have on pain and organ function. Finally, published morbidity data are presented from clinical trials that have compared general with regional analgesia in an attempt to demonstrate any benefit of either technique, and so to promote much needed research and audit into perioperative morbidity.

Pathophysiology of pain

The pain experienced after abdominal and thoracic surgery is generally agreed to be the most severe in man and multiple afferent somatic and visceral pathways are involved in the transmission of nociceptive information. For example the somatic nerves involved after upper abdominal surgery are bilateral and include the lower six intercostal nerves, the ilioinguinal and iliohypogastric, the phrenic and the upper four lumbar nerves.[2] The viscera derive their nerve supply from the right and left vagi (parasympathetic) and the splanchnic nerves (T5-12) which form the coeliac plexus (sympathetic).[2]

Most nociceptive signals from the thoracoabdominal viscera travel through afferent fibres in the sympathetic nerves. Parasympathetic fibres contain only afferents concerned with visceral function.[3] Quantitatively visceral afferents are greatly outnumbered by somatic afferents.[4] Noxious stimuli to the GI tract appear to be detected by small numbers of non-specific visceral receptors which project to viscerosomatic neurones in the spinal cord over several segments and in some cases through long supraspinal loops.[4] Moreover, there is a widespread functional divergence of information within the spinal cord. Thus, the conscious appreciation of somatic pain involves activation of pathways normally concerned with integration of cutaneous impulses, and can be blocked largely by modulation of activity within the substantia gelatinosa. Once visceral nociceptive pathways are activated, widespread effects ensue because of the extensive functional divergence of polysynaptic networks.[5] Impulses in non-myelinated C fibres result in poorly localized diffuse dull pain which is associated with reflex somatic and autonomic activity and sympathetic outflow. This is quite unlike the sharp precise concentrated quality of somatic pain. The results are more prolonged and difficult to control. Attempts at peripheral blockade of one of these pathways will not inhibit the response at spinal cord level because the other afferent pathways will have been activated. Similar complex pathways exist in the innervation of the thorax and pelvis.

The effects of pain on organ function

Postoperative major organ function is to a large degree influenced by pain and the associated increase in autonomic activity. When there is no 'fight flight or fright' situation, as after elective surgery, the changes are largely deleterious.

Cardiovascular

The physiological effects of noradrenaline, adrenaline and dopamine on the heart and circulation are well known but, to summarize, tachycardia and increased contractility both result in increased myocardial work and oxygen consumption. In the presence of increased systemic vascular resistance these may cause myocardial ischaemia and infarction especially if there is pre-existing disease. Decreased organ blood flow, most notably to the liver and kidneys, may also result in ischaemia and cell necrosis. Adrenaline has been shown, in animal studies, to increase pulmonary arterio-venous shunting due to non-uniform vasodilatation/constriction within the pulmonary vasculature and both alpha and beta blockade can reduce this.[6, 7] During cardiac catheterization there is a close correlation between pulmonary vascular resistance and pulmonary artery catecholamine concentrations in the presence of pulmonary arterial hypertension.[8] Local neurogenic stimuli have also been noted to contribute to the pulmonary platelet trapping seen in shock.[9]

Respiratory

It has been known for many years that, particularly after abdominal and thoracic procedures, reflexes through sympathetic pathways result in substantial inhibition of normal breathing patterns.[10] Furthermore, studies have demonstrated that even in the virtual or complete absence of pain, pulmonary function remains depressed for many days following surgery.[11]

Among those other factors known to influence pulmonary function are diaphragmatic contractility, abdominal distension, secondary ileus, age, size, type of surgery and incision, personality, pre-existing lung disease, smoking habits, neuromuscular disease and muscle weakness, changes in thoracoabdominal blood volume and, of considerable importance, the position of the patient.[12, 13]

Pain itself leads to a reduction in both static and dynamic lung parameters, most notably functional residual capacity (FRC) and peak flow rate.[14] Basal atelectasis occurs rapidly and results in hypoxia, hypercapnia, and venous admixture.

Pain also decreases tidal volume and the ability to breathe deeply so that the ability to cough is impaired.[15] Thus secretions are retained and airways collapse so providing an ideal environment for sepsis. This in turn further enhances the metabolic response to trauma which increases catecholamine synthesis.

Gastrointestinal

Catecholamines have potentially harmful effects on gastrointestinal blood flow and function. In hypovolaemic states splanchnic blood flow is greatly decreased and healing may be compromised in patients with gastrointestinal anastomoses.[16] The GI tract plays a central role in protein catabolism after injury.[17] Mucosal cell atrophy may occur secondary to ischaemia and hypoxia so resulting in breakdown of the gut barrier to micro-organisms and endotoxin, further stimulating the glucocorticoid response and immunosuppression. Intestinal secretions and sphincter tone are increased whilst motility is decreased. Thus, gastric dilatation and paralytic ileus are believed to be caused by local sympathetic inhibitory reflexes both within the gut wall and the spinal cord.[18] A similar state occurs within the genitourinary tract resulting in acute retention of urine.

Renal

Postoperatively the effects of circulating catecholamines, adrenergic stimulation, hypotension, hypoxia and the neuroendocrine response (i.e. renin, angiotensin II, aldosterone, and ADH) on renal function are well recognized.[3] In addition, enkephalins, kinins and prostaglandins PGE2 and PG1 (prostacyclin) have important vasodilator actions. PGE2 is further stimulated by ADH, atrial natriuretic peptide and Ag II, making the overall extrinsic control of renal vessels complex. Although intrinsic autoregulation is more important than these extrinsic factors in maintaining renal blood flow, care must be taken in the postoperative period to minimize their effects.

Metabolic

Catecholamines, particularly adrenaline, promote the catabolic state increasing blood sugar, plasma lactate and free fatty acid (FFA). In addition, adrenaline contributes to the retention of sodium and water and excretion of potassium, while fluid shifts from the extracellular to vascular and intracellular compartments are also mediated partly by catecholamines. By inhibiting pancreatic release of insulin and antagonizing its peripheral effects on glucose utilization, adrenaline inhibits anabolism, promoting a negative nitrogen balance.[19–21]

In addition to the catecholamines, several substances are released in response to trauma which, although partly beneficial, are also known to have potentially detrimental effects on the well-being of the patient. Of these, the most important are cortisol, glucagon, histamine and interleukin 1. In the presence of severe trauma or sepsis these disturbances can lead to rapid depletion of lean body mass and organ failure.[22].

Although the above changes are well documented little is known about the trigger mechanisms. Pain itself is not one of these but will amplify the effects. Afferent stimuli travelling through nociceptive and autonomic pathways play an important role, particularly in clean, uncontaminated surgery. In addition, haemorrhage, acidosis, hypoxia, infection, anxiety and heat loss amplify the response.[22] Histamine, serotonin, bradykinin and substance P are released locally in response to nociceptive stimuli. Prostaglandins and interleukins can also modulate many of the observed responses.[23]

Immunofunction

Our understanding of the mechanisms which initiate postoperative immunosuppression is also poor but the magnitude of the trauma, and presumably the pain, directly correlates with both serum cortisol and the degree of immunosuppression.[24] Indeed this suppression has also been implicated in the formation of tumour metastases and postoperative sepsis.[25] After tumour resection there is down-regulation of the cellular immune system and T-helper lymphocytes are decreased causing an imbalance between these and the suppressor lymphocytes.[26] After major surgery both helper and suppressor cells are suppressed and in addition circulating numbers of natural killer (NK) cells, which have a wide range of cytotoxic activity, particularly against tumour cells, are depressed.[27] Thus cellular immunity is disturbed for up to seven days postoperatively and changes in the above plasma parameters persist for much longer.[25]

The release of histamine may initiate some of these changes since the release of interleukin II, itself a pivot in the release of both lymphocyte subpopulations and humoral responses[28] has been shown to involve H2 receptors on the releasing macrophages.[29] Indeed studies have confirmed the beneficial effects of IV ranitidine on the postoperative decrease in delayed cutaneous hypersensitivity which is a manifestation of lymphocyte suppression.[30]

Psychological

Pain whilst difficult to define is readily understood by all who experience it. Its effects on the individual patient's psyche will therefore be determined by many factors. These include race, religion, age, sex, social circumstance and upbringing, fear, anxiety and neurosis, time of day, marital status, the presence or absence of relatives and friends, the expectations of the patient prior to operation and the nature, site and extent of the surgery performed. Philips and Cousins[5] highlighted the need to relieve anxiety and to maintain normal sleep patterns throughout the perioperative period. Sleep can be disrupted by many factors, but predominantly pain, for up to 48 hours after surgery. In this regard premedication with benzodiazepines such as temazepam and lorazepam are said to have least effect on normal sleep patterns. Few would deny that the psychology of pain is largely neglected in the perioperative period. Various therapies have been used to reduce psychological trauma, particularly the placebo effect and counselling of the patient before and after surgery.

Influences of analgesic drugs

It is important now to consider the actions and side-effects of the three available classes of analgesics used most commonly to control postoperative pain.

Opioid analgesia

All opioid drugs, regardless of the route of administration, act on receptors widely and unevenly dispersed in the central nervous system. Several distinct types of receptors have been described including mu, delta, kappa and sigma. The theoretical advantage of pure kappa agonists and mixed agonist/antagonists in minimizing respiratory depression has not yet been evaluated in humans but animal studies are encouraging.[31]

Descending control of pain transmission has been shown to originate in the cortex and reticular formation and the predominant transmitters appear to be noradrenaline, serotonin and enkephalins.[32] Systemic opioids owe their efficacy to activation of these systems.

Problems with systemic opioids
It has been consistently demonstrated that postoperative patients seldom receive sufficient analgesia from this method. The underlying reasons for this include insufficient knowledge of relevant physiology and pharmacology by attendant staff, uniform prescriptions, acceptance of sub-maximal analgesia by senior staff, fear of side-effects and fear of addiction.

Much can be done to prevent some of these doubts and misconceptions by increasing the quality and quantity of teaching of the subject. 'PRN' prescriptions deserve special attention in this context since there are several diverse reasons for a patient requesting analgesia (or not!), and also for the nursing staff to further delay administration. *This leads to prolonged periods of breakthrough pain.* Pain is, whatever else, a predominantly miserable experience and should ideally be treated on a prophylactic, or curative basis, at regular intervals in the initial postoperative period, taking care to avoid overdose in debilitated patients. At present PRN prescriptions merely provide disinterested senior colleagues with a safety valve for harassed junior members of staff.

A basic understanding of pharmacodynamics and pharmacokinetics is somewhat of a prerequisite for rational pain treatment with systemic opioids. This has, however, failed to solve the practical problem of safe, predictable, effective and simple analgesia, because intramuscular administration leads to a considerable range of both serum concentrations and clinical response (for the same operation), and again prolongs periods of breakthrough pain due to slow absorption.

Intravenous regimes may therefore seem a more rational approach. Predictable, stable and controlled analgesic serum levels can theoretically be achieved using nomograms and multivariate equations, but such data have only been obtained for patient-controlled techniques. Cessation of an intravenous infusion will result in rapid decline in serum levels but this is not the case for intramuscular injections.

Side-effects

The main side-effects of opioid administration *regardless of the route* are respiratory depression, drowsiness (which may or may not be desirable), nausea and vomiting, hypotension, constipation and pruritis.

When effective amounts of opioids are administered there is a direct dose-dependent depression of the medullary respiratory centre so that the CO_2 response curve is flattened and shifted to the right. Effects are seen within 2–5 minutes of intravenous administration, 30 minutes of intramuscular injections and 1–½ hours after subcutaneous administration.[33] The effect may last several hours. The risk of delayed respiratory depression after spinal administration is probably in the region of 0.5 per cent.[34] It may occur as late as 15 hours after epidural morphine and is thought to be due to a rostral spread of the opioid within the CSF. Thus, continuous surveillance of patients for this length of time is advisable.

The effects on gastrointestinal function are described in more detail later but, to summarize, they may in the postoperative period precipitate or exacerbate regurgitation, nausea, vomiting and paralytic ileus. Anti-emetics are an invariable adjunct to these agents and may add to the drowsiness or dysphoria of the patient (which may or may not be a desirable goal) in any given situation.

Hypotension occurs as a result of both central depression of vasomotor tone and peripheral release of histamine,[35] and is frequently seen. There is a strong correlation between plasma histamine levels and haemodynamic changes, which partly explains the relative cardiovascular stability of the newer agents such as fentanyl and sufentanil over morphine and pethidine. In any event, the lowered blood pressure can be effectively remedied by simple measures.

Pruritis may prove troublesome, particularly with epidural administration (see later in this chapter). Cough suppression is commonly seen with all agents and may result in retention of sputum and inhaled secretions predisposing to chest infection. Retention of urine occurs in about 30 per cent of patients regardless of the route of administration and, finally, small doses of opioids may actually raise plasma noradrenaline and adrenaline concentrations by sympathetic stimulation.[33]

Local anaesthetics

The mode of action of these drugs is discussed elsewhere.

The choice of drug at present is somewhat empirical and operator-dependent, but bupivacaine has a clear advantage where intermittent boluses are given because of its longer duration of action and its relatively sparing effect on motor fibres. If a continuous technique is used duration of drug action is not important. Systemic toxicity, though not common, should be borne in mind and better agents with a more selective action sought. The value of adding adrenaline to the solution to improve the quality of the block remains controversial. With regard purely to quality of postoperative analgesia, continuous epidural local anaesthesia, when indicated, is better than any other single agent technique.

Side-effects of central block
The most frequent side-effects of central nerve block are hypotension, motor paralysis and urinary retention.

Hypotension occurs predominantly as a result of sympathetic blockade and cardiac output will decrease if the block is too high, vagal overactivity exists or concomitant cardiac depressant drugs are given as well. If necessary, treatment is by an intramuscular or intravenous injection of vasopressor, oxygen, head-down tilt and increased intravenous fluids. Atropine will relieve bradycardia due to vagal overactivity. It is vital to remember that:

1. Pre-existing hypovolaemia must always be treated prior to epidural local anaesthetic administration.

2. Hypotension in a postoperative patient may be due to haemorrhage and a high index of suspicion must guard against this being overlooked.

Urinary retention is probably the only significant side-effect when epidural anaesthesia is used for lower limb surgery. It occurs frequently with all types of epidural sometimes necessitating catheterization. However, most major surgery is covered by a broad-spectrum antibiotic as prophylaxis against bacteraemia and sepsis.

Motor blockade may be unpleasant for the patient and delay mobilization but may be decreased by using a lower concentration and the smallest possible dose. There will still be a significant action on smaller A-delta and C fibres. Local anaesthetic toxicity as a result of an inadvertent overdose or intravascular injection occurs infrequently whilst haematoma and abscess formation are extremely rare.

The regression of sensory level of blockade and pain relief with time is another practical hurdle associated with prolonged postoperative use of local anaesthetic.[36] Too few studies have been performed to correctly elicit the underlying mechanism(s) but the addition of an opioid to the infusion helps prevent this decline in effect with time.[37]

Other nerve blocks
Intercostal nerve blockade has begun to wane in popularity as a single dose procedure, but continuous blockade of several intercostal segments using a single catheter and extrapleural spread of local anaesthetic may prove valuable once the necessary data have been collected. The data now available on the use of an interpleural catheter have confirmed that it can be an extremely effective means of analgesia[38-41] but intraperitoneal[42] and intravenous local anaesthesia[43] are ineffective. Incisional bupivacaine places no additional demands on nursing staff and, since side-effects are few, merits further consideration.

Non-steroidal anti-inflammatory drugs (NSAIDs)

These drugs inhibit the enzyme cyclo-oxygenase which controls the synthesis of prostaglandins, prostacyclins and thromboxanes, all of which are inflammatory mediators at the site of injury or trauma (some, e.g. paracetamol, also inhibit this enzyme within the CNS).

They are most effective in treating minor degrees of pain. Those which may be given parenterally may be as effective in relieving pain of a severe nature. Other potential advantages are their antipyretic and antiplatelet activities, and the latter may be of use in the prevention of thrombo-embolism. However, all NSAIDs have a high number of side-effects,[44] particularly affecting the gastrointestinal tract and coagulation, and all individual drugs are implicated. However, ibuprofen (Brufen) would appear to be the safest in this regard[45] and, when used in suppository form, it may further reduce the incidence of gastrointestinal side-effects.

Except when asthma, peptic ulcer, and bleeding dyscrasias are present, an NSAID such as ibuprofen may be recommended for baseline analgesia in patients undergoing surgery. It may be argued that they could be given prophylactically with the premedication and continued for at least 24 hours. The apparent synergism between NSAIDs, opioids and regional anaesthesia requires further research.

The effects of analgesics on pain

The opioids

No matter how these drugs are administered systemically, analgesia remains poor[46, 47] and the most notable response of patients to questioning is that they are in no pain provided that they lie still and make no attempt to cough or move. Because both of these activities are important in the prevention of venous thromboembolism, basal atelactasis and chest infections, this is not ideal. Systemic administration remains the standard with which all other techniques of pain relief are compared, but this has consistently been shown to be less effective than epidural or spinal administration. Indeed studies have also shown that parenteral NSAIDs are as good as systemic opioids in certain types of pain.[48–50]

When pain is assessed by the visual analogue scale from 0–10 (0 = no pain, 10 = the worst possible) most patients will have scores ranging from 6–10 without analgesia and these can be reduced to between 3–6 with systemic opiates. Pain scores at least less than four would appear a desirable figure and it is most curious that barely a handful of all the studies performed on postoperative pain have attempted to assess the effects of mobilization and coughing on pain scores.

In 1985 it was demonstrated that the administration of IV morphine could re-establish the original level of blockade after epidural bupivacaine had begun to regress.[51] This was thought to be a consequence of activation of descending inhibitory pathways and led to an increase in the use of combined anaesthetic/opioid in the epidural space. The resulting analgesia has been shown to be superior in quality and duration.

The use of very low volume infusions of bupivacaine and diamorphine via thoracic epidural has been advocated. Whilst a considerable advantage over the administration of systemic opioids, pain relief is not total and supplementary analgesics are required. Indeed, high infusion concentrations of this combination, compared with interpleural bupivacaine alone, demonstrated no significant differences in the additional need for morphine or in pain scores between the two groups.[38]

Regional anaesthesia

Virtually every known local anaesthetic technique has been used by single dose, intermittently, or by continuous infusion, to provide anaesthesia/analgesia after thoracic or abdominal surgery. Only the intraperitoneal and intravenous routes would appear to afford no benefit to the patient either in terms of analgesia or reduced morphine requirements.[42, 43] The effectiveness of wound instillation is unconfirmed,[52–56] but proper attention to anatomic detail may resolve the situation because large muscle splitting incisions are difficult to infiltrate accurately. Toxicity is the only worrying side-effect, because improved local perfusion secondary to vasodilatation and the bacteristatic action of local anaesthetics balance the concern that wound instillation may predispose to infection.

Specific blockade of the nerves supplying the area of incision using the intercostal, interpleural or paravertebral techniques further improves the quality of analgesia because somatic wound pain is the most important component of postoperative pain. However, total analgesia is not produced in the majority of cases, presumably due to failure to block visceral afferent pathways and spinal reflexes. There is understandable concern that these techniques may result in pneumothorax, and repeated intercostal blocks are not to be recommended. There is a risk of pneumotharax at the time of insertion of intercostal, interpleural and paravertebral catheters but the overall incidence is small, and further reduced with experience and meticulous attention to detail.

All of these techniques are variations on the theme of segmental anaesthesia designed to decrease the incidence of local anaesthetic toxicity and avoid the complications of epidural or spinal anaesthesia. For upper abdominal surgery using a unilateral incision, they compare favourably with thoracic epidural block.[42, 57] However, once again visceral reflexes are not obtunded by any of these techniques and total pain relief is therefore not achieved. The use of thoracolumbar anaesthesia can provide total pain relief particularly when a combined opioid/local anaesthetic mixture is used.

NSAIDs

These are extremely effective in the management of musculoskeletal pain. Because somatic pain is the major component of postoperative pain they have been shown to be effective in its management.[58, 59] They have also been shown to be as effective as opioids in the management of visceral pain such as renal colic,[49] are of considerable benefit in the management of dysmenorrhoea and have been shown to have a morphine-sparing effect after upper abdominal surgery.[60] Whilst side-effects are protean during prolonged administration they should not be a problem if the use of NSAIDs is restricted to the first few days after surgery.

Effects of analgesia

Cardiovascular

The Opioids
These may occasionally cause severe hypotension as a consequence of arterial and venous dilatation either by alpha adrenergic blockade or by histamine release. In addition to these actions pethidine with its atropine-like activity results in higher heart rates than the other drugs.[35]

Fentanyl and methadone are said to have the least depressant effect on myocardial contractility of the opioids but data from controlled human studies are few.

Regional Anaesthesia

The effects of central and paravertebral blockade on the sympathetic nerves may produce changes in cardiovascular function. Such techniques should not be instituted in shocked patients and only used with great care when severe haemorrhage is a high risk. Other than this the effects of sympathectomy will be largely advantageous and the changes produced will be determined by the height of the block. Other factors which will modify these effects on the cardiovascular system include the reduction of pain and a direct action of local anaesthetics on the myocardium and brain stem.

The sympathetic innervation of the heart is from T1–T5 through the middle cervical, stellate and first four thoracic ganglia. Stimulation increases both heart rate and contractility. The same segments supply vasoconstriction fibres to the upper limbs while the legs are supplied by T10 to L2. The adrenal medulla is supplied from T8 to L1, the abdominal viscera from T6–L2, liver T7–T9 and the kidneys from T10–L1.[61] Whilst somatic sensory blockade is usually detectable at a higher dermatomal level than motor blockade during epidural blockade, the height of sympathetic blockade is controversial. As assessed by changes in skin temperature, one study showed the sympathetic block to be up to six segments higher than the sensory block.[62] Bromage has suggested that sympathetic block is incomplete at all levels and thus the cardiovascular effects of spinal and epidural anaesthesia may involve much more subtle cardiovascular changes than one would expect from the upper level of sensory blockade.[15] However, for clinical purposes the subdivision into high (above T6) and low (below T6) blockade is sufficient for a basic understanding of their effects. The most obvious consequence of a low block is hypotension due to vasodilatation and increased regional perfusion, but when the block is high decreased cardiac output will predispose to hypoperfusion.[63] For example, thoracolumbar blockade produced by two separate injections of 1% mepivacaine (at C7–T1 and L3–4) resulted in small, but significant decreases in CVP, cardiac index, heart rate, stroke volume, blood pressure and peripheral resistance.[64] Epidural 2% lignocaine with a sensory block from T2–T12 produced no deleterious changes in the circulation.[65] Indeed, cardiac output was maintained in the presence of a decreased systemic vascular resistance so that LV work decreased by 14 per cent. Finally, epidural block from T4–L4 with 2% lignocaine produced no significant change in cardiac output in the presence of a decreased mean arterial pressure, increased lower limb flow and reduced upper limb flow.[65]

These effects were observed in patients without pain. The analgesic and sympathetic effects of epidural block have been shown to have a beneficial effect on cardiovascular function after cholecystectomy in otherwise healthy individuals by decreasing afterload and 0_2 requirements, and reducing heart rate so improving coronary perfusion and myocardial oxygenation.[65] Similar results were obtained with thoracic epidural anaesthesia.[66] In morbidly obese patients undergoing gastric bypass, oxygen requirements and left ventricular stroke work were again decreased by thoracic epidural anaesthesia.[67] Systemic hypertension often follows coronary artery and aortic surgery, presumably as a result of stimulation of the sympathetic system and adrenal medulla. Following coronary artery surgery thoracic epidural lidocaine 1% decreased preload and afterload and raised the ratio of diastolic time/systolic time thus improving the balance between myocardial oxygen demand and delivery.[68] Systolic arterial pressure was significantly lower using epidural block when compared with an opioid infusion.[69]

The NSAIDs
No data are available regarding the cardiovascular effects of NSAID-analgesia. Obviously regional blood flow will be subject to subtle control from the various prostaglandins but overt alterations of cardiac output and systemic vascular resistance have not been described.

Respiratory effects

The opioids
Pain acts as a respiratory stimulant counteracting the respiratory depression of opioids, but this effect will disappear when analgesia is effective. Opioids act via μ-receptors in the medulla to produce hypoventilation by decreasing both tidal volume and respiratory rate, thus exacerbating the respiratory effects of pain. Furthermore, morphine has been shown to preferentially depress the rib cage contribution to tidal volume.[70] There is no evidence that any of the currently available agonists differ in their ability to produce these effects, but drugs with pure κ-agonist properties may prove advantageous.

In patients undergoing elective upper abdominal surgery, studies have repeatedly shown that there is a decrease of approximately 60 per cent from the preoperative figures for peak flow rate (PFR), forced expiratory volume in the first second (FEVI) and forced vital capacity (FVC) while functional residual capacity (FRC), is decreased by 30 per cent.[14] These parameters can take up to 14 days to return to normal. Because of its association with small airways closure it is generally agreed that FRC is the single most important lung parameter influencing hypoxaemia and postoperative pulmonary complications, although by inhibiting coughing, restrictive falls in PFR, FEV, and FVC will also be significant.[71]

In addition to their adverse effects on ventilation, systemic opioids interact with sleep patterns to produce profound episodic oxygen desaturation due to airway obstruction or apnoea in the postoperative period.[72] Cough suppression will also predispose to retention of secretions.

Regional anaesthesia

While regional anaesthetic techniques have been shown to be of clear benefit in the reduction of postoperative pulmonary dysfunction they may themselves contribute to, and confuse, the picture. Intercostal muscle paralysis and lack of effect on the inhibition of contractility of the diaphragm may decrease efficacy. Cervical and high thoracic epidural anaesthesia using 2% mepivacaine have produced a 20–30 per cent decrease in FRC, VC, FEV_1 and total lung capacity within 30 minutes.[73] High thoracic epidural (T1–T5) with 0.5% bupivacaine achieved similar but less pronounced results.[74] However, several studies on unpremedicated patients with no pulmonary disease have failed to demonstrate any significant alteration in ventilation and FRC with both spinal and epidural anaesthesia to T4.[75]

Intercostal nerve block appears to afford some improvement in FEV_1; FVC and PEFR when used for unilateral abdominal incisions but not for midline incisions.[76] Incisional infiltration appears to have little if any effect.[55] Interpleural paravertebral and thoracic epidural block also have varying effects[38, 57] but appear superior to conventional systemic opioids[77] Intraperitoneal instillation of bupivacaine has no effect.[42] The combination of epidural bupivacaine and morphine does not produce better pulmonary function than that achieved with bupivacaine alone, despite improving analgesia.[37]

NSAIDs

There are few data on the use of NSAIDs and postoperative pulmonary dysfunction. By preventing vasoconstriction and platelet plugging mediated by arachnidonic acid metabolites, NSAIDs might decrease shunting, but properly controlled studies have not been performed. The combination of epidural bupivacaine and morphine with systemic indomethacin did not significantly alter the clinical picture.[1]

Gastrointestinal system

By increasing sympathetic activity, pain, *per se*, will increase intestinal secretions and smooth muscle tone and decrease intestinal motility.[5] These changes are believed to be due to inhibitory reflexes within the gut wall and within the spinal cord which project to bulbar centres.[78] Gastric dilatation will ensue and may result in regurgitation which increases the risk of an aspiration pneumonia. The last section of the bowel to resume normal motility is the colon.[79] Paralytic ileus itself leads to increased intra-abdominal pressure so compromising pulmonary function and further increasing the risk of aspiration. Distension will further contribute to the patient's level of discomfort.

Opioids

The administration of opioids will exacerbate this picture by direct actions on both the chemoreceptor trigger zone and the GI tract. In addition they decrease resting pressure at the lower oesophageal sphincter,[84] increase gastric antral pressure and duodenal smooth muscle tone, and decrease gut peristalsis.[33] Animal studies have suggested that epidural fentanyl may inhibit reflexes that result in postoperative ileus[80] but a combined epidural regime of bupivacaine and morphine after upper abdominal surgery did not produce this effect[81] Morbidly obese patients given epidural morphine after gastroplasty showed an increase in gastric contents but a paradoxical reduction in bowel stasis.[82] Finally in normal volunteers epidural morphine delayed gastric emptying.[83]

Regional anaesthesia

Epidural local anaesthesia has beneficial effects on most gastrointestinal parameters. Thus, different studies have demonstrated no change in lower oesophageal sphincter pressure,[84] enhanced gastric emptying,[85] increased stomach and small bowel electrical activity,[86] increased small and large bowel flood flow[87] (particularly within the anastomotic area) and, if infusions are continued for 48 hours, a decrease in large bowel transit time.[88, 89] Intraperitoneal instillation of bupivacaine has been shown to shorten the period of colonic inhibition after cholecystectomy, thought to be a result of a direct action on intramural inhibitory reflexes.[90]

NSAIDs

NSAIDs have been used successfully in the management of visceral pain since a decrease in prostaglandin activity will decrease smooth muscle spasm. However, research on the postoperative use of these drugs is still in progress and no data are available on their effects on GI function. The risk of GI bleeding and stress ulceration should be considered before prescribing these drugs.

Renal system

Little is known about the specific effects of opioids on postoperative renal function except that they increase ADH secretion thus increasing the neuroendocrine effects on the kidney.[35]

Neural blockade influences fluid and electrolyte balance by several mechanisms. Hypotension secondary to sympathetic blockade decreases glomerular filtration rate and the secretion of aldosterone, cortisol catecholamines, renin and ADH. Renal reflex pathways controlling tubular transport rates are blocked. Furthermore, studies have suggested that post-traumatic anuria may be reversed by neural blockade.[22] Despite these clear differences between opioids and neural blockade the overall evidence for or against any beneficial effect of either technique is inconclusive for reasons similar to those relevant to the metabolic effects (see below) and because fluid management is so variable.

The use of NSAIDs has been shown to have detrimental effects on renal function by toxic, idiosyncratic and ischaemic mechanisms.[91] This latter is thought to be due to a reduction in the synthesis of PGE2 decreasing medullary blood flow. Thus their use should at present be avoided in any patient known to have pre-existing renal impairment.

Immunocompetence

The development of sepsis, wound and systemic, is undoubtedly one of the major contributing factors to surgical morbidity. The development of prophylactic antibiotic policies has contributed to the gradual decline in the overall incidence in the past twenty years but specific types of surgery, most notably thoracic and colonic, continue to carry a high risk. Prosthetic surgery also has serious consequences if the prosthesis becomes infected. In the presence of sound surgical technique, asepsis and antibiotic prophylaxis, the most likely explanation for an infective episode would seem to be the immunosuppression which occurs postoperatively and persists for at least four to five days or even longer in patients with malignant disease.[25] Immunocompetence is a multicomponent mechanism involving non-specific, humoral and cellular components, and changes are predominantly correlated with the magnitude of the surgery. General anaesthesia *per se* has no significant effect.[24] Because systemic opioids are known to cause significant release of histamine and induce immunosuppression in animal studies,[92] much work has to be done to clarify whether or not this contributes to the overall state of immunosuppression seen in the postoperative patient. Epidural fentanyl has not been shown to have any beneficial effect on reduced T-cell function postoperatively.[93]

Again there is little information regarding the use of NSAIDs alone, but they have been shown to prevent postoperative pyrexia (since this is mediated by prostaglandin E2) when used with epidural bupivacaine.[94] Apart from the aforementioned beneficial effect of IV ranitidine on T-cell function[30] the only method available at present to modify postoperative immunosuppression is regional anaesthesia. After lower abdominal procedures, continuous epidural analgesia, which blocks the stress response completely, modifies different aspects of the immune response. However, continuous epidural anaesthesia for upper abdominal surgery failed to modify perioperative activity of NK cells in spite of a partial inhibition of the stress response.[24] During epidural blockade with 2% mepivacaine the degree of complement activation during aortic surgery was less pronounced when compared with general anaesthesia.[95]

No data are available regarding the incidence of wound infection but a so-called 'wash-out effect' has been claimed using wound infiltration with local anaesthetic.[56] Both peripheral and central neural blockade will result in sympathetic denervation and, presumably, in an increased blood flow and oxygen delivery, enhancing wound healing and decreasing sepsis. Against these arguments is the concern that complete absence of pain will result in over-exertion during the convalescent period and increase the risk of dehiscence. No study has specifically addressed these issues.

Metabolic influences of analgesia

As has been stated previously the stress response to lower abdominal surgery may be blocked by spinal or epidural anaesthesia. In contrast to lower abdominal surgery, studies that have been performed on the stress response after upper abdominal surgery are inconclusive. High dose opioid infusions will obtund the intraoperative Stress response but are not practicable in the postoperative setting for obvious reasons. Patient-controlled systemic opioid analgesia following cholecystectomy causes a moderate reduction in the cortisol response.[96] Combining opioids with local anaesthetics improves the quality and duration of analgesia but produces no further effect on the stress response.[97] The addition of systemic indomethacin did not further modify the glucose and cortisol responses to cholecystectomy.[1] However, studies have suggested that postoperative nitrogen losses can be decreased if NSAIDs are commenced before surgery.[98] Sympathoadrenal stimulation is reduced in most studies, the adrenocortical response appearing to be more difficult to suppress. These studies have all employed 0.5% bupivacaine as the main analgesic but some have used it in combination with other local anaesthetic agents or morphine. Recent work with evoked potentials has suggested that it does not produce as effective a block as had been believed previously,[99, 100] but there are no data comparing the local anaesthetics. Paravertebral and intercostal catheters can reduce the sympathoadrenal response[101, 102] but intraperitoneal[42] and interpleural[38] local anaesthetics have no effect.

Problems with the differences between the various studies include poor documentation of the spread of anaesthesia obtained with the concomitant degree of analgesia, and whether this was maintained throughout the study, for there are real problems with regression of the block. Since pain is clearly a contributory factor to the degree of the stress response, future studies should make such details quite clear when describing the technique.

Duration of analgesia also differs between the studies, the most marked modifications in the stress response being achieved with prolonged infusions and extensive blockade; paradoxically, perhaps the best designed of all these studies failed to show any effect of 72 hours combined epidural bupivacaine plus morphine on any measured parameter.[97] Different surgical procedures are included in some studies and, clearly, the combination of abdominal and thoracic procedures does not allow exact interpretation.[103]

Two other aspects of methodology are worthy of mention. Firstly, some studies do not exactly describe the intravenous fluid regimens used. Secondly, there may be ethnic and cultural differences in the stress response to trauma. Studies have been performed worldwide and there are several differences in the results, with the most strikingly positive effects being reported from Japan.[98, 104–106]

There are three main reasons why the responses to upper abdominal and thoracic procedures are so difficult to block. Firstly, there is the diffuse nature of the regional somatic and visceral nerve supply. Secondly, the greatest bulk of the sympathetic nervous system is within the thoracolumbar region of the spinal cord. Thus, somatic and visceral nociception will be maximal when this region is directly stimulated. Thirdly, and perhaps most importantly, the volume and concentration of drug used for thoracic blockade are significantly less than for lumbar blockade.

Postoperative morbidity and the choice of analgesia

The remainder of this chapter summarizes data from controlled clinical studies that have compared postoperative complications in patients who have received regional anaesthesia with postoperative complications in patients that have received general anaesthesia (GA) plus systemic opioid analgesia. In most of the studies patients receiving regional anaesthesia (RA) were also given a general anaesthetic during surgery.

Cardiac morbidity

As stated earlier there is good evidence that the perioperative demands on the heart are decreased by RA probably because of the diminished catecholamine response to surgery. In a series of 45 patients undergoing urgent major vascular surgery within three months of myocardial infarction, epidural anaesthesia resulted in significantly better intraoperative stability than general anaesthesia.[131] Postoperative re-infarction (1/23 vs 5/22) and death from myocardial infarction (1/23 vs 3/22) were less in the RA group but the differences were not statistically significant. Another study on high-risk patients compared RA with GA in thoracic, abdominal or vascular procedures and the incidence of postoperative cardiovascular failure was significantly reduced by the epidural regimen.[111] Studies looking specifically at perioperative ECG changes show an insignificant reduction in the incidence of ischaemic changes with RA.[107, 114, 118, 120, 132, 133]

Pulmonary morbidity

Although epidural analgesia seems to be better than other regimens in minimizing the pulmonary effects of surgery postoperatively, few studies have compared the incidence of pulmonary infections with the choice of anaesthetic. Several authors confuse atelectasis, which is of questionable importance, with pneumonia. Thus whilst the incidence of atelectasis is decreased by regional anaesthesia in most of the comparative studies[77, 81, 107–121, 123–125], only three have shown regional anaesthesia to be of clear clinical benefit on the incidence of pulmonary infection. This was after cholecystectomy,[113] lower limb vascular surgery[122] and thoracic, abdominal or vascular procedures in high-risk patients respectively.[111] The use of wound infiltration or intercostal blockade on postoperative pulmonary complications is probably of no clinical value, since the published data have shown conflicting results.[52, 126–130]

Gastrointestinal morbidity

Regardless of the apparently clear advantage of regional anaesthesia over general for colonic surgery the only prospective trial to date failed to demonstrate a decreased incidence of anastomotic dehiscence.[134] The study employed a 'high spinal' technique established after the induction of GA, thus neither the height nor the duration of the block were determined. Furthermore, both study groups received systemic opioid before and after surgery thereby confusing the overall clinical picture. When epidural bupivacaine was compared with intramuscular pentazocine for colonic surgery there was a highly significant reduction in the transit time of barium, and the time to pass both flatus and faeces.[78] Similarly, postoperative epidural bupivacaine when compared with epidural morphine, each given for 42 hours, reduced the duration of ileus following hysterectomy by more than half (22 hours vs. 56 hours).[83]

There have been three documented instances of either intraoperative or immediate postoperative anastomotic dehiscence under regional anaesthesia.[135, 136] These cases hardly justify the recommendation that elective colonic surgery be a contra-indication to the use of regional anaesthesia. In these cases the increased colonic activity probably served to expedite the diagnosis of poor surgical technique at a time when the patient's condition remained optimal. Furthermore it has been recognized for many years that central block is relatively contra-indicated in the patient with an acute abdomen.

Blood loss and thromboembolism

With the growing concern regarding both the transmission of AIDS and the development of tumour recurrence after blood transfusion, any technique which can minimize perioperative blood loss is to be recommended. One of the arguments against the use of NSAIDs is that they may increase perioperative bleeding as a result of dose-dependent inhibition of platelet function. There is little information regarding this but what is available does not lend support to the theory.[58] Because subcutaneous heparin is used widely as prophylaxis and not considered to increase blood loss, a controlled study comparing their relative efficacies on the incidence of thromboembolism would appear important. It has been clearly established that embolic phenomena can be prevented in patients with chronic cardiovascular disease treated with long-term aspirin.[137]

The relationship between induced hypotension and blood loss is not clear, although this is the explanation commonly given for the effect of central neural blockade. A recent prospective controlled study on patients undergoing total hip replacement showed that under epidural anaesthesia, mean arterial pressure, mean pulmonary arterial pressure, right atrial pressure and peripheral venous pressure were all significantly decreased.[138] From this it was deduced that decreased blood loss was probably a result of diminished venous oozing.

Studies on upper abdominal procedures under thoracic or lumbar epidural anaesthesia have failed to show any significant reduction although the amount of transfused blood was lower.[81, 104, 139–142] However one study of patients undergoing cholecystectomy showed a significant 50 per cent reduction in intraoperative blood loss in the epidural group.[133] Controlled studies looking at a variety of lower abdominal, vascular and orthopaedic procedures all demonstrate significant reductions in blood loss[116, 122, 138, 143–157, 173] except for the operation of transurethral prostatectomy in one study where the reduction is not significant.[145]

Coagulation and fibrinolysis are profoundly altered following surgery, the ability to coagulate increasing whilst fibrinolysis, after initial enhancement, is subsequently decreased. These changes appear to be only slightly dependent on neurogenic or adrenal hormone stimulation.[22] Despite this, RA may have a beneficial effect by decreasing platelet aggregation and blood viscosity,[155, 157] preserving endothelial structure and greatly enhancing lower limb blood flow.[22, 158]

A highly significant reduction in the incidence of thromboembolism is also seen after operations below the umbilicus when RA is employed.[144, 149–151, 159–161] Similarly, the incidence of pulmonary embolism as assessed by perfusion lung scanning was significantly lower in patients receiving RA as opposed to GA.[150, 151]

In three of four studies performed after upper abdominal surgery[133, 139, 140] no difference was found in the incidence of thromboembolism but these patients were given thoracic as opposed to lumbar epidural blockade and the limits of the block were not clearly defined. Sympathetic blockade and thereby increased flow to the lower limbs will only occur if the block involves the L1 and L2 spinal nerves. The fourth study[81] was unique in that DVT prophylaxis was given to the control group but not to the epidural group, and showed that lumbar epidural anaesthesia alone was as effective as subcutaneous heparin. As yet, only one study has been performed combining RA with other forms of DVT prophylaxis. Addition of epidural analgesia did not further reduce the incidence of leg thromboembolism or positive pulmonary scintigrams in patients receiving antithrombotic treatment with dextran 70 after hip surgery.[154]

Cerebral function

Despite the commonly held belief that mental performance is less affected by RA, the available data on this subject are conflicting.[107, 109, 110, 115, 116, 122, 162–165] Furthermore the mechanisms which lead occasionally to prolonged mental deterioration after surgery have not been elucidated. It would appear that anaesthesia does not initiate this deterioration but no study has addressed the contribution of opioid analgesia postoperatively despite the well-recognized CNS effects of these drugs. It is generally believed that, in elderly patients, it is the admission to hospital itself rather than the surgery that is important.[166] A recent study has highlighted the importance of the preoperative use of anticholinergic drugs and a history of depression in precipitating confusion.[109] Finally intraoperative hypocarbia and postoperative hypoxia and electrolyte imbalance have also been implicated in the aetiology.[166]

Convalescence and hospital stay

In a study comparing local infiltration of lignocaine with general anaesthesia for short stay inguinal hernia the RA group could walk, eat and pass urine significantly earlier but the discharge rate at 24 hours was similar.[167] Another study comparing a low-dose continuous combined morphine and bupivacaine regime with both systemic opioids and three other epidural regimens after abdominal surgery, showed that this combined regimen provided superior pain relief and significantly improved mobilization postoperatively.[168]

Postoperative mobilization and length of hospital stay has also been reduced by RA in 8 of 10 studies[52, 107, 111, 114, 117, 118, 120, 126, 145, 169] but this has only achieved statistical significance in one.[118] It should be further emphasized that these studies combine a variety of surgical procedures and anaesthetic techniques and thus no conclusion may be drawn. The time for mobilization following hip surgery was reduced in two of three studies.[110, 118, 169]

No comparative data exist for postoperative fatigue, muscle performance, return to work, etc. The development of the postoperative fatigue syndrome seems to be related to a diminished ability of the cardiovascular system to adapt to the increased demands of the operative stress.[170]

Summary

What conclusions can be drawn from the foregoing to positively influence future clinical practice? The discussion has been based on four main issues. Firstly, that current postoperative analgesic practice is a 'cruel and callous disgrace'[171] and needs both a change in attitude and in emphasis before improvements can be made. With regard to major thoracoabdominal surgery, analgesia can only be improved upon by blocking sympathetic as well as somatic pathways since these contribute enormously to the observed effects of surgery. Secondly, as a consequence, regional anaesthesia in all its various forms is a great improvement on systemic morphine analgesia and should be used more often. This having been said, these techniques carry their own inherent morbidity, no less important than that of morphine analgesia but, equally, no more dangerous since any inherent danger of such a technique would be readily discernible in a controlled study. Not one of the controlled studies performed has demonstrated a significantly greater morbidity with regional anaesthesia over general anaesthesia plus systemic opioid.

Thirdly, with the growing use of NSAIDs as an option for major surgery the current use of systemic opioids as the first choice for severe postoperative pain falls well short of requirements with regard both to efficacy and side effects. Perhaps they should now be given a place alongside other available options rather than continue to enjoy widespread unrivalled popularity as the 'drug of choice'. All well controlled studies published to date indicate that the degree of pain relief obtained with a single agent is not always adequate, and combinations of drugs give much superior results. A mixture of opioid and a local anaesthetic given epidurally together with an NSAID given enterally or parenterally provides a three-pronged attack on nociception, each component of which acts at a different site. Analgesia is thereby enhanced while the dose of each drug can be substantially decreased compared to that needed when used alone.

The incidence and severity of serious side-effects, particularly respiratory depression and hypotension, should be considerably reduced.

The final issue is whether or not the neuroendocrine response is important for the well-being of the patient after planned elective surgery. Certainly, if prolonged, as for example in the case of postoperative sepsis, it would indeed appear to be detrimental to body mass and tissue reserve. Roisen has argued a case for perioperative sympathectomy based on the improved postoperative course of cardiac surgical patients using beta-blocking agents.[172] The use of alpha- and beta-blocking agents may be important in this respect. However reflex changes are not prevented or reduced and catecholamine release is still high. There are good reasons why both cortisol and catecholamine release should be prevented or at least minimized in the hope of reducing the incidence of sepsis and maintaining homeostasis. 'Stress-free' anaesthesia is not a new concept and should not be regarded as separate from current anaesthetic practice but it does require a different approach in postoperative nursing and medical care.

If by the siting of a single catheter it is possible to offer *inter alia* complete afferent neural blockade resulting in relief of pain, abolition of the stress response, efferent sympathetic blockade resulting in increased blood flow to the region of the blockade, the avoidance of respiratory depression and hypoxia, DVT prophylaxis and a reduced susceptibility to infection, then such a technique should be more widely advocated and efforts made to overcome its avoidable side-effects.

References

1. Schulze S., Roikjaer O., Hasselstrom L., Jensen N. H., Kehlet H., Epidural bupivacaine plus morphine plus systemic indomethacin eliminates pain but not systemic response and convalescence after cholecystectomy. *Surgery* 1988; **103**: 321–7.
2. Last R. J. *Anatomy: Regional and Applied*. Edinburgh: Churchill Livingstone, 1978.
3. Ganong W. F. *Review of Medical Physiology*, 12th Edition. Los Altros, California: Lange Medical Publications, 1985.
4. Cervero F. *Phil. Trans. R. Soc. Lond.* 1985; **308**: 325–37.
5. Phillips G. D., Cousins M. J. Neurological mechanisms of pain and the relationship of pain anxiety and sleep. In: Cousins M. J., Phillips G. D. (Eds). *Acute Pain Management*, Melbourne: Churchill Livingstone, 1986.
6. Berk J. L. Hagen J. F., Koo R. Pulmonary insufficiency caused by epinephrine. *Ann. Surg.* 1973; **178**: 423.
7. Berk J. L. Hagan J. F., Koo R. Effect of alpha and beta adrenergic blockade on epinephrine induced pulmonary insufficiency. *Ann. Surg.* 1976; **183**: 369–76
8. O'Neill M. J., Pennock J. L., Seaton J. F., Dortimer A. C., Waldhausen J. A., Harrison T. S. Regional endogenous plasma catecolamine concentrations in pulmonary hypertension. *Surgery*. 1980; **84 (1)**: 140–6.

9. Thorne L. J., Kuenzig, McDonald H. M., Schwartz S. I. Effect of denervation of a lung on pulmonary platelet trapping associated with traumatic shock. *Surgery* 1980; **88 (2)**: 208–14.
10. Guenter C. A. Toward prevention of postoperative pulmonary complications. *Am. Rev. Respir. Dis.* 1984; **130**: 4–5.
11. Benhamou D., Samii K., Noviant Y. Effect of analgesia on respiratory muscle function after upper abdominal surgery. *Acta Anaesthesiol. Scand.* 1983; **27**: 22–5.
12. Syndow F. W. The influence of anaesthesia and postoperative analgesic management on lung function. *Acta Chir. Scand.* Suppl. 550, 1988; 159–168.
13. Hedenstierna G. Mechanisms of postoperative pulmonary dysfunction. *Acta Chir. Scand.* Suppl. 550, 1988; 152–8.
14. Craig D. B. Postoperative recovery of pulmonary function *Anesth. Anal.* 1981; **60**: 46–52.
15. Bromage P. R. *Epidural Analgesia.* Philadelphia: W. B. Saunders, 1978.
16. Tagart R. E. B. Colorectal Anastomosis: factors influencing success. *J. R. Soc. Med.* 1981; **74**: 111–8.
17. Wilmore D. W. Alterations in protein, carbohydrate and fat metabolism in injured and septic patients. *J. Amer. Coll.* Nutr. 1983; **2**: 3–13.
18. Furness J. B., Costa M. Adynamic ileus, its pathogenesis and treatment. *Med. Biol.* 1974; **52**: 82–9.
19. Frayn K. N. Hormonal control of metabolism in trauma and sepsis. *Clinical Endocrinology* 1986; **24**: 577–99.
20. Little R. A., Frayn K. N. (eds). *The scientific basis for the care of the critically ill.* Manchester University Press: 1985.
21. Wilmore D. W., Smith R. J., O'Dwyer S. T., Jacobs D. O., Ziegler, T. R., Wang X. D. The Gut: a central organ after surgical stress. *Surgery* 1988; **104**: 917–23.
22. Kehlet H. Modification of responses to surgery by neural blockade: clinical implications. In: Cousins M. J., Bridenbaugh P. O. (Eds.) *Neural blockade in clinical anesthesia and management of pain.* 2nd Ed. J. B. Lippincott, Philadelphia: 1987.
23. Dinarello C. A. Interleukin–1. *Reviews of Infectious Diseases* 1984; **6**: 51–94.
24. Tonnesen E. Immonulogical aspects of anesthesia and surgery. *Danish Med. Bull.* 1989; **36**: 263–81.
25. Lennard T. W. J., Shenton B. K., Bortotta A. et al. The influence of surgical operation on components of the immune system. *Br. J. Surg.* 1985; **72**: 771–6.
26. Hole A., Bakke O. T-lumphocytes and the subpopulations of T-helper and T-suppressor cells measured by monoclonal antibodies (T11, T4 and T8) in relation to surgery under epidural and general anaesthesia. *Acta Anaesthesiol. Scand.* 1984; **28**: 296–300.
27. Tonnesen E., Huttel M. S., Christensen N. J., Schmitz O. Natural killer cell activity in patients undergoing upper abdominal surgery: relationship to the endocrine stress response, *Acta Anaesthesiol. Scand.* 1984; **28**: 654–60.
28. Fletcher M., Goldstein A. L. Recent advances in the understanding of the biochemistry and clinical pharmacology of Interleukin-2. *Lymphokine Res.* 1987; **6**: 45–57.

29. Beer D. J., Rocklin R. E. Histamine-induced suppressor-cell activity. *J. All. Clin. Immunol.* 1987; **72**: 439–52.
30. Nielsen H. J. Ranitidine for prevention of postoperative suppression of delayed hypersensitivity. *Am. J. Surg.* 1989; **157**: 291–4.
31. Althous J. S., von Voigtlander P. F. Difamo C. A., Miller E. D. Effect of U-5)488H, a selective k-analgesic on the minimum alveolar concentration of halothane in the rat. *Anesth. Analg.* 1987; **66**: 391–4.
32. Cousins M. J., Mather L. E. Intrathecal and epidural administration of opioids. *Anesthesiology* 1984; **61**: 276–310.
33. Duthie D. J. R., Nimmo W. S. Adverse effects of opioid analgesic drugs. *Brit. J. Anaesth.* 1987; **59**: 61–77.
34. Gustafsson L. L, Schildt B., Jacobsen K. Adverse effects of extradural and intrathecal opiates. Reports of a nationwide survey in Sweden. *Brit. J. Anaesth.* 1982; **54**: 479–85.
35. Bovill J. G., Sebel P. S., Stanley T. H. Opioid analgesics in Anaesthesia: with special reference to their use in cardiovascular anaesthesia. *Anesthiology* 1984; **61**: 731–55.
36. Bigler D., Lund C., Mogensen T., Hjortso N. C., Kehlet H. Tachyphylaxis during postoperative epidural analgesia–new insights. *Acta Anaesthesiol. Scand.* 1987; **31**: 664–5.
37. Hjortso N. C., Lund C., Mogensen T., Bigler D., Kehlet H. Epidural morphine improves pain relief and maintains sensory analgesia during continuous epidural bupivacaine after abdominal surgery. *Anesth. Analg.* 1986; **65**: 1033–6.
38. Scott N. B., Mogensen T., Bigler D., Kehlet H. Comparison of continuous intrapleural vs. epidural administration of 0.5% bupivacaine on pain, metabolic response and pulmonary *Acta Anaesthesiol. Scand.* 1989; **33**: 535–9.
39. Seltzer J. L., Larijani G. E., Goldberg M. E., Marr A. T. Intrapleural bupivacaine – a kinetic and dynamic evaluation. *Anesthesiology* 1987; **67**: 798–800.
40. Vadeboncouer T. R., Riegler F. X., Fautt R. S., Weinberg G. L. A randomised double-blind comparison of the effects of interpleural bupivacaine and saline on morphine requirements and pulmonary function after cholecystectomy. *Anesthesiol.* 1989; **71**: 339–43.
41. Brismar B., Pettersson N., Tokics L., Strandberg A., Hedenstlerna G. Postoperative analgesia with intrapleural administration of bupivacaine-adrenaline., *Acta Anaesthesiol. Scand.* 1987; **31**: 515–20.
42. Scott N. B., Mogensen T., Greulich A., Hjortso N. C., Kehlet H. No effect of continuous intraperitoneal bupivacaine on analgesia pulmonary function and the postoperative stress response. *Brit. J. Anaesth.* 1988; **61**: 165–8.
43. Birch K., Jorgensen J., Chraemmer Jorgensen H., Kehlet H. Effect of 1V lignocaine on pain and endocrine-metabolic responses after surgery. *Brit. J. Anaesth.* 1987; **59**: 721–4.
44. C. S. M. Update – Non-steroidal anti-inflammatory drugs and serious gastrointestinal adverse reactions – 1. B. M. J. 1986; **292**: 614.
45. C. S. M. Update – Non-steroidal anti inflammatory drugs and serious gastrointestinal adverse reactions – 2. B. M. J. 1986; **292**: 1190–1.
46. Rosenberg P. H., Heino A., Scheinin B. Comparison of intramuscular analgesia, intercostal block, epidural morphine and on-demand IV

fentanyl in the control of pain after upper abdominal surgery. *Acta Anaesthesiol. Scand.* 1984; **28**: 603–7.

47. Ellis R., Haines D., Shah R., Cotton B. R., Smith G. Pain relief after upper abdominal surgery – a comparison of IM morphine, ublingual buprenorphine and self-administered IV pethidine. *Br. J. Anaesth.* 1982; **54**: 421–7.

48. Mattila M. A. K., Ahlstrom-Bengs E., Pekkola P. Intravenous indomethacin or oxycodone in prevention of postoperative pain. *B. M. J.* 1983; **287**: 1026.

49. Uden P., Rentzhog L., Berger T. A comparative study on the analgesic effects of indomethacin and hydromorphine chloride – atropine in acute ureteral stone pain. *Acta Chir. Scand.* 1983; **149**: 497–9.

50. Cashman J. N., Jones R. M., Foster J. M. G., Adams A. M. Comparison of infusions of morphine and lysine acetylsalicylate for the relief of pain after surgery. *Br. J. Anaesth.* 1985; **57**: 255–8.

51. Lund C., Mogensen T., Hjortso N. C., Kehlet H. Systemic morphine enhances spread of sensory analgesia during postoperative epidural bupivacaine infusion. *Lancet* 1985; **ii**: 1156–7.

52. Patel M. J., Lanzafame R. J., Williams J. S., Mullen B. V., Hinshaw, J. R. The effect of incisional infiltration of bupivacaine hydrochloride upon pulmonary function atelectasis and narcotic requirement following elective cholecystectomy. *Surg. Gyn. Obst.* 1983; **157**: 338–40.

53. Sinclair R., Cassuto J., Hogstrom S. et al. Topical anaesthesia with lidocaine aerosol in the control of postoperative pain. *Anesthesiology* 1988; **68**: 895–901.

54. Egan T. M., Hjerman S. J., Doucette E. J., Normand S. L., McLeod R. S. A randomised controlled trial to determine the effectiveness of fascial infiltration of bupivacaine in preventing respiratory complications after elective abdominal surgery. *Surgery* 1988; **104**: 734–40.

55. Gibbs P., Purushotham A., Auld C., Cuschieri R. J. Continuous wound perfusion with bupivacaine for postoperative wound pain. *Brit. J. Surg.* 1988; **75**: 923–4.

56. Thomas D. F. M. Lambert W. G., Lloyd-Williams K. The direct perfusion of surgical wounds with local anaesthetic solution: an approach to postoperative pain? *Ann. R. Coll. Surg. Engl.* 1983; **65**: 226–9.

57. Bigler D., Dirkes W., Hansen R., Rosenberg J., Kehlet H. Effects of thoracic paravertebral block with bupivacaine versus combined thoracic epidural block with bupivacaine and morphine on pain and pulmonary function. *Acta Anaesthesiol. Scand.* 1989; **33**: 561–4.

58. Reasbeck P. G., Rice M. L., Reasbeck J. C. Double-blind controlled trial of indomethacin as an adjunct to narcotic analgesia after major abdominal surgery. *Lancet* 1982; ii 115–7.

59. Owen H., Glavin R. J., Shaw N. A. Ibuprofen in the management of postoperative pain. *Brit. J. Anaesth.* 1986; **58**: 1371–5.

60. Gillies G. W. A., Kenny G. N. C., Bullingham R. E. S., McArdle C. S. The morphine-sparing effect of ketorolac: A study of a new parenteral non-steroidal anti-inflammatory agent after upper abdominal surgery. *Anaesthesia* 1987; **42**: 727–31.

61. Warwick R., Williams (Eds). *Gray's Anatomy*. 35th British Ed. Philadelphia: Saunders, 1973.

62. Chamberlain D. P., Chamberlain B. D. L. Changes in skin temperature

of the trunk and their relation to sympathetic blockade during spinal anaesthesia. *Anesthesiology* 1986; **65**: 139–43.

63. Covino B. G., Scott D. B., *Handbook of Epidural Anaesthesia and Analgesia.* Copenhagen: Schultz Medical Information APS, 1985.

64. McLean BA. P. H., Mulligan G. W., Otton P. et al. Haemodynamic alterations associated with epidural anaesthesia. *Surgery* 1967; **62**: 79–87.

65. Sjogren S., Wright B. Circulatory changes during continuous epidural blockade. *Acta Anaesthesiol. Scand. Supp.* 1972; **46**: 5–25.

66. Holmdahl M. H., Sjorgen S., Strom G. et al. Clinical aspects of continuous extradural blockade for postoperative pain relief. *Uppsala J. Med. Sci.* 1972; **77**: 47–56.

67. Gelman S., Laws H. L., Potzick J., Strong S., Smith L., Erdemir H. Thoracic epidural vc. balanced anaesthesia in morbid obesity. An intraoperative and postoperative study. *Anesth. Analg.* 1980; **59**: 902–8.

68. Hoar P. F., Hickey R. F., Ullyot D. J. Sustemic hypertension following myocardial revascularisation. A method of treatment using epidural anaesthesia. *J. Thorac. Cardiovasc. Surg.* 1976; **71**: 859–64.

69. Kumar B., Hibbert G. R. Control of hypertension during aortic surgery using lumbar epidural blockade. *Brit. J. Anaesth.* 1984; **56**: 797.

70. Rigg J. R. A., Rondi P. Changes in rib cage and diaphragm contribution to ventilation after morphine. *Anesthesiology* 1981; **55**: 507–14.

71. Engberg G. Factors influencing the respiratory capacity after upper abdominal surgery. *Acta Anaesthesiol. Scand.* 1985; **29**: 434–45.

72. Catley D. M., Thornton C., Jordan C. Lehane J. R., Royston D., Jones J. G. Pronounced episodic oxygen desaturation in the postoperative period: its association with ventilatory pattern and analgesic regimen. *Anesthesiology* 1985; **63**: 20–8.

73. Takasaki M., Takahashi T. Respiratory function during cervical and thoracic extradural analgesia in patients with normal lungs. *Brit. J. Anaesth.* 1980; **52**: 1271–5.

74. Sundberg A., Wattwil M., Arvill A. Respiratory effects of high thoracic epidural anaesthesia. *Acta Anaesthesiol. Scand.* 1986; **30**: 215–7.

75. Bowler G. M. R., Wildsmith J. A., Scott D. B. Epidural administration of local anaesthetics. In: Eds. Cousins, M. J., Phillips, G. D., *Acute Pain Management. Clinics in Critical Care Medicine.* Edinburgh: Churchill Livingstone, 1986; 187–235.

76. Crawford R. D., Thompson G. E., Intercostal Block. In: Cousins M. J., Phillips, G. D. (Eds.). *Acute Pain Management.* Melbourne: Churchill Livingstone, 1986.

77. Hendolin H., Lahtinen J., Lansimies E., Tuppurainen T., Partanen, K. The effect of thoracic epidural analgesia on respiratory function after cholecystectomy. *Acta Anaesthesiol. Scand.* 1987; **31**: 645–51.

78. Ahn H., Bronge A., Johansson K., Ygge H., Lindhagen J. Effect of continuous postoperative epidural analgesia on intestinal motility. *Brit. J. Surg.* 1988; **75**: 1176–8.

79. Aitkenhead A. R. Anaesthesia and bowel surgery. *Brit. J. Anaesth.* 1984; **56**: 95–101.

80. Lisander B., Stenqvist O. Extradural fentanyl and postoperative ileus in rats. *Brit. J. Anaesth.* 1981; **53**: 1237–8.

81. Hjortso N. C., Neumann P., Frosig et al. A controlled study on the effect of epidural analgesia with local anaesthetics and morphine on morbidity

after abdominal surgery. *Acta Anaesthesiol. Scand.* 1985; **29**: 790–6.

82. Rawal N., Sjostrand U., Christoffersen G., Dahlstrom B., Arvill A., Rydman H. Comparison of intramuscular and epidural morphine for postoperative analgesia in the grossly obese: influence on postoperative ambulation and pulmonary function. *Anesth. Analg.* 1984; **63**: 583–92.

83. Thoren T., Sundberg A., Wattwil M., Garvill J. G., Jorgensen U. Effects of epidural bupivacaine and epidural morphine on bowel function and pain after hysterectomy. *Acta Anaesthesiol. Scand.* 1989; **33**: 181–5.

84. Thoren T., Carlsson E., Sandmark S., Watwil M. Effects of thoracic epidural analgesia with morphine or bupivacaine on lower oesophageal sphincter pressure: an experimental study in man. *Acta Anaesthesiol. Scand.* 1988; **32**: 391–4.

85. Nimmo W. S., Littlewood D. G., Scott D. B., Prescott L. F., Gastric emptying following hyperectomy with extradural analgesia. *Brit. J. Anaesth.* 1978; **50**: 559–61.

86. Gelman S., Freigenberg Z., Dintzman M., Levy E. Electroenterography following cholecystectomy. *Arch. Surg.* 1977; **112**: 580–4.

87. Johansson K., Ann H., Lindhagan J., Tryselius U. Effect of epidural anaesthesia on intestinal blood flow. *Brit. J. Surg.* 1988; **75**: 73–6.

88. Ahn H., Lindhagen J., Bronge A., Ygge H. The effect of postoperative epidural local anaesthetics on gastro-intestinal motility. *5th Congress European Society of Regional Anaesthesia*, Malmo, Sweden 1986 (abstract).

89. Scheinin B., Asantila R., Orko R. The effect of bupivacaine and morphine on pain and bowel function after colonic surgery. *Acta Anaesthesiol. Scand.* 1987; **31**: 161–4.

90. Rimback G., Cassuto J., Faxen A., Hogstrom S., Wallin G., Tollesson P. O. Effect of intraabdominal bupivacaine instillation on postoperative colonic motility. *GUT* 1986; **27**: 170–5.

91. Kincaid-Smith P. Effects of non-narcotic analgesics on the kidney. *Drugs* 1986; **32 (Suppl. 4)**: 109–28.

92. Tubaro E., Borelli G., Croce C., Cavallo G., Santiangelli C. Effect of morphine on resistance to infection. *J. Inf. Diseases* 1983; **148**: 656–66.

93. Hjortso N. C., Andersen T., Frosig F., Neumann P., Rogon E., Kehlet H. Failure of epidural analgesia to modify postoperative depression of delayed hypersensitivity. *Acta Anaesth. Scand.* 1984; **28**: 128–131.

94. Schultze S., Schierbeck J., Sparso B. H., Bisgaard M., Kehlet H. Influence of neural blockade and indomethacin on leukocyte temperature and acute phase protein response to surgery. *Acta Chir. Scand.* 1987; **153**: 255–9.

95. Bengtson A., Lannsjo W., Heidman M. Complement and anaphylotoxin responses to cross clamping of the aorta. *Brit. J. Anaesth.* 1988; **61**: 160–4.

96. Moller I. W., Dinesen K., Sondergard S., Knigge U., Kehlet H. Effect of patient controlled analgesia on plasma catecholamines cortisol and glucose after cholecystectomy. *Brit. J. Anaesth.* 1988; **61**: 160–4.

97. Hjortso N. C., Christensen N. J., Andersen T. et al. Effects of the extradural administration of local anaesthetics and morphine on the urinary excretion of cortisol catecholamines and nitrogen following surgery. *Brit. J. Anaesth.* 1985; **57**: 400–3.

98. Asoh T., Shirasaka C., Uchida I., Tsuji H. Effects of indomethacin on endocrine responses and nitrogen loss after surgery. *Ann. Surg.* 1987; **206**: 770–6.

99. Lund C., Hansen O. B., Mogensen T., Kehlet H. Effect of thoracic epidural bupivacaine on somatosensory evoked potentials after dermatomal stimulation. *Anesth. Analg.* 19897; **66**: 731–4.

100. Lund C., Selmar P., Hansen O. B., Kehlet, H. Effect of intrathecal bupivacaine on somatosensory evoked potentials due to dermatomal stimulation. *Anesth. Analg.* 1987; **66**: 809–13.

101. Giesecke K., Hamberger B., Jarnberg P. O., Klingstedy C. Paravertebral block during cholecystectomy: effects on circulatory and hormonal responses. *Brit. J. Anaesth.* 1988; **61**: 652–6.

102. Pither C. E., Bridenbaugh L. D., Reynolds F., Perioperative intercostal block: effect on the endocrine metabolic response to surgery. *Brit. J. Anaesth.* 1988; **60**: 730–2.

103. Bromage P. R., Shibata H. R., Willoughby H. W. Influence of prolonged epidural blockade on blood sugar and cortisol responses to operations upon the upper part of the abdomen and thorax. *Surg. Gynecol. Obstet.* 1971; **132**: 1051–6.

104. Tsuji H., Shirasaka C., Asoh T., Takeuchi Y. Influences of splanchnic nerve blockade on endocrine metabolic responses to upper abdominal surgery. *Brit. J. Surg.* 1983; **70**: 437–9.

105. Tsuji H., Shirasaka C., Asoh T., Ushida I. Effects of epidural administration of local anaesthetics or morphine on postoperative nitrogen loss and catabolic hormones. *Brit. J. Surg.* 1987; **74**: 421–5.

106. Tsuji H., Shirasaka C., Asoh T., Takeuchi Y. Influences of splanchnic nerve blockade on endocrine metabolic responses to upper abdominal surgery. *Brit. J. Surg.* 1983; **70**: 437–9.

107. Racle J. P., Benkhadra A., Poy J. Y., Gleizal B., Gaudray A. Etude comparative de l'anaesthésie générale et de la rachianesthésia chez la femme âgée dans la chirurgie de la hanche. *Ann. Fr. Anesth. Reanim* 1986; **5**: 24–30.

108. White I. W. C., Chappell W. A., Anaesthesia for surgical correction of fractured femoral neck. A comparison of three different techniques. *Anesthesia* 1980; **35**: 1107–10.

109. Berggren D., Gustafson Y., Eriksson et al. Postoperative confusion following anaesthesia in elderly patients with femoral neck fractures. *Anaesth. Analg.* 1987; **66**: 497–504.

110. Bigler D., Adelhoj B., Petring O. U., Pedersen N. O., Busch P., Kalhke P. Mental function and morbidity after acute hip surgery during spinal and general anaesthesia. *Anaesthesia* 1985; **40**: 672–6.

111. Yeager M. P., Glass D. D., Neff R. K., Brinck-Johnsen T. Epidural anaesthesia and analgesia in high-risk surgical patients. *Anesthesiology* 1987; **66**: 729–36.

112. Spence A. A., Smith G. Postoperative analgesia and lung function. A comparison of morphine with extradural block. *Brit. J. Anaesth.* 1971; **43**: 144–8.

113. Cuschieri R. J., Morran C. G., Howie J. C., McArdle C. S. Postoperative pain and pulmonary complications: comparison of three analgesic regimes. *Brit. J. Surg.* 1985; **72**: 495–8.

114. Hendolin H. The influence of continuous epidural anaesthesia on the peri- and postoperative course of patients subjected to retropubic prostatectomy. Thesis, University of Kuopio, Finland, 1980.

115. Hole A., Terjesen T., Breivik H. Epidural vs. general anaesthesia for

total hip arthroplasty in elderly patients. *Acta Anaesthesiol. Scand.* 1980; **24**: 279–87,

116. Mann R. A. M., Bissett W. I. K. Anaesthesia for lower limb amputation. *Anaesthesia* 1983; **38**: 1185–91.

117. Miller L., Gertel M., Fox G. S., McLean L. D. Comparison of effect of narcotic and epidural analgesia on postoperative respiratory function. *Am. J. Surg.* 1976; **131**: 291–4.

118. Pflug A. E., Murphy T. M., Butler S. H., Tucker G. T. The effects of postoperative peridural analgesia on pulmonary therapy and pulmonary complication. *Anesthesiology* 1974; **1**: 8–17.

119. McLaren A. D., Stockwell M. C., Reid V. T. Anaesthetic techniques for surgical correction of fractured neck of femur. A comparative study of spinal plus general anaesthesia in the elderly. *Anaesthesia* 1978; **33**: 10–4.

120. Tolksdorff W., Raiss G., Streibel J-P., Lutz H. Intra- and postoperative kardiopulmonale komplikationen bei transurethralen prostatrareseketionen in intubationsnarkose und ruckenmarksnaher leitungsanasthesie. In Wust H. J., Zindler, M. (Eds). *Neue Aspekte in der Regional Anasthesie I,* Berlin: Springer Verlag, 1980; 146–160

121. Addison N. V., Brear F. A., Budd K., Whittaker M. Epidural anaesthesia following cholecystectomy. *Brit. J. Surg.* 1974; **61**: 850–2.

122. Cook P. T., Davis M. J., Cronin K. D., Moran P. A prospective randomised trial comparing spinal anaesthesia using hyperbaric cinchocaine with general anaesthesia for lower limb vascular surgery. *Anaesth. Intens. Care* 1986; **14**: 373–80.

123. Jayr C., Mollie A., Bourgain J. L. et al. Postoperative pulmonary complications: general aesthesia with postoperative paravertebral morphine compared with epidural analgesia. *Surgery* 1988; **104**: 57–63.

124. Logas W. G., El-Baz N., El-Ganzouri A., et al. Continuous thoracic epidural analgesia for postoperative pain relief following thoracotomy: a randomised prospective study. *Anesthesiol.* 1987; **67**: 787–91.

125. Hasenbos M., Van Egmond J., Bielen M., Crul J. F. Postoperative analgesia by high thoracic epidural versus intramuscular nicomorphine after thoractotomy – Part III. *Acta Anaesthesiol. Scand.* 1987; **31**: 608–15.

126. Crawford E. D., Skinner D. G. Intercostal nerve block with thoracoabdominal and flank incisions. *Urology* 1982; **14**: 25–8.

127. Delilkan A. E., Lee C. K., Yong N. K Ong S. C., Ganendran A Postoperative local analgesia for thoracotomy with direct bupivacaine intercostal blocks. *Anaesthesia* 1973; **28**: 561–7.

128. Levack I. D., Holmes J. D., Robertson G. S. Abdominal wound perfusion for the relief of postoperative pain. *Brit. J. Anaesth.* 1986; **58**: 615–9.

129. Ross W. B., Tweedie J. H., Leong Y. P., Wyman A., Smithers B. M., Does intercostal blockade improve patient comfort after cholecystectomy? *Brit. J. Surg.* 1987; **74**: 63.

130. Baxter A. D., Jonnings F. O., Harris R. S., Flynn J. F., Way J. Continuous intercostal blockade after cardiac surgery. *Brit. J. Anaesth.* 1987; **59**: 162–6.

131. Reiz S., Balfors E., Sorensen M. B. et al. Coronary haemodynamic effects of general anaesthesia and surgery. Modification by epidural analgesia in patients with ischaemic heart disease. *Reg. Anesth.* 1982; **7**: S8.

132. Couderc E. F., Mauge F., Duvaldstrein P., Desmonts J. M. Results

comparatifs de l'anesthésie générale et peridurale chez le grand viellard dans la chirurgie de la hanche. *Anesth. Analg Reanim* 1977; **34**: 987–97.

133. Hendolin H., Lahtinen J., Lansimiues E., Tuppurainen T. The effect of thoracic epidural analgesia on postoperative stress and morbidity. *Annales Chirurgiae et Gynaecologiae* 1987; **76**: 234–40.

134. Worsley M. H., Wishart H. Y., Peebles-Brown D. A., Aitkenhead, A. R. High spinal nerve block for large bowel anastomosis. A prospective study. *Brit. J. Anaesth.* 1988; **60**: 336–40.

135. Bigler D., Hjortso N. C., Kehlet H. A case of disruption of colonic anastomosis two hours postoperatively during continuous epidural analgesia. *Anaesthesia* 1985; **40**: 278–80.

136. Treissman D. A. Disruption of colonic anastomosis associated with epidural anaesthesia. *Reg. Anesth.* 1980; **5**: 22–3.

137. Anti-platelet trialists' collaboration. Secondary prevention of vascular disease by prolonged anti-platelet therapy. *Brit. Med. J.* 1988; **296**: 320–31.

138. Modig J. Beneficial effects on blood loss in total hip replacement when performed under lumbar epidural anaesthesia versus general anaesthesia. An explanatory study. *Acta Chir. Scand. Suppl. 550,* 1988; 95–103.

139. Hendolin H., Tupparainen T., Lahtinen J. Thoracic epidural analgesia and deep venous thrombosis in cholecystectomised patients. *Acta Chir. Scand.* 1982; **148**: 405–0.

140. Mellbring G., Dahlgren S., Reiz S., Sunnegarfh O. Thromboembolic complications after major abdominal surgery: effect of thoracic epidural analgesia. *Acta Chir. Scand.* 1983; **149**: 263–8.

141. Rutberg H., Hakanson E., Anderberg B., Jorfedlt L., Martensson J., Schildt B. Effects of the extradural administration of morphine or bupivacaine on the endocrine response to upper abdominal surgery. *Brit. J. Anaesth.* 1984; **56**: 233–8.

142. Traynor C., Paterson J. L., Ward L. D., Morgan M., Hall G. M. Effects of extradural analgesia and vagal blockade on the metabolic and endocrine response to upper abdominal surgery. *Brit. J. Anaesth.* 1982; **54**: 319–23.

143. Blunnie W. P., McIlroy P. O. W., Merrett J. D., Dundee J. W., Cardiovascular and biochemical evidence of stress during major surgery associated with different techniques of anaesthesia. *Brit. J. Anaesth.* 1083; **55**: 611–8.

144. Hendolin H., Mattila M. A. K., Poikalainen E. The effect of lumbar epidural analgesia on the development of deep venous thrombosis of the legs after open prostatectomy. *Acta Chir. Scand.* 1981; **147**: 425–9.

145. McGowan S. W., Smith G. F. N. Anaesthesia for transurethral prostatectomy. *Anaesthesia* 1980; **35**: 847–53.

146. Jakobsen B. W., Pedersen J., Egebjerg B. B. Postoperative lymphocytopenia and leucocytosis after epidural and general anaesthesia. *Acta Anaesthesiol. Scand.* 1986; **30**: 668–71.

147. Keith I. Anaesthesia and blood loss in total hip replacement. *Anaesthesia* 1977; **32**: 440–50.

148. Hole A., Unsgaard G., Breivik H. Monocyte functions are depressed during and after general but not epidural anaesthesia. *Acta Anaesthesiol. Scand.* 1982; **26**: 301–7.

149. Modig J., Hjelmstedt A., Sahlstedt B., Maripuu E. Comparative influences of epidural and regional anaesthesia on deep venous thrombosis

and pulmonary embolism after total hip replacement. *Acta Chir. Scand.* 1981; **147**: 125–30.

150. Modig J., Borg T., Karlstrom G., Maripuu E., Sahlstedt B. Thromboembolism after total hip replacement. Role of epidural and general anaesthesia, *Anesth. Analg.* 1983; **62**: 174–80.

151. Modig J., Maripuu E., Sahlstedt B. Thromboembolism following total hip replacement. A prospective investigation of 94 paitents with emphasis on efficacy of lumbar epidural anaesthesia in prophylaxis. *Reg. Anesth.* 1986; **11**: 72–9.

152. Chin S. P., Abou Madi M. N., Witvoet J., Montagne J. Blood loss in total hip replacement. Extradural v. phenoperidine analgesia. *Brit. J. Anaesth.* 1982; **54**: 491–5.

153. Davis F. M., McDermott E., Hickton C. et al. Influence of spinal and general anaesthesia on haemostasis during total hip arthroplasty. *Brit. J. Anaesth.* 1987; **59**: 561–71.

154. Fredin H., Rosberg B. Anaesthetic techniques and thromboembolism in total hip arthroplasty. *Eur. J. Anaesth.* 1986; **3**: 273–81.

155. Henny C. P., Odoom J. A., Tencate J. W. et al. Effects of extradural bupivacaine on the haemostatic system. *Brit. J. Anaesth.* 1986; **58**: 301–5.

156. Modig J., Karlstrom G. Intra and postoperative blood loss and haemodynamics in total hip replacement when performed under lumbar epidural versus general anaesthesia. *Eur. J. Anaesthesiol.* 1987; **4**: 345–55.

157. Borg T. Modig J. Potential antithrombotic effects of local anaesthetics due to their inhibition of platelet function. *Acta Anaesthesiol. Scand.* 1985; **29**: 739–42.

158. Cousins M. J., Wright C. J. Graft muscle skin blood flow after epidural block in vascular surgical procedures. *Surg. Gynecol. Obstet.* 1971; **133**: 59–64.

159. Davis F. M., Laurenson V. G. Spinal anaesthesia or general anaesthesia for emergency hip surgery in elderly patients. *Anaesth. Intens. Care* 1981; **9**: 352–8.

160. McKenzie P. J., Wishart H. Y., Gray I., Smith G., Effect of anaesthetic technique on deep vein thrombosis. *Brit. J. Anaesth.* 1985; **57**: 853–7.

161. Davis F. M., Laurenson V. G., Gillespie W. J., Wells J. E., Foate J. Newman E. Deep Vein thrombosis after total hip replacement. A comparison between spinal and general anaesthesia. *J. Bone Joint Surg. (BR)* 1989; **71**: 181–5.

162. Karhunen V., Jonn G. A comparison of memory function following local + general anaesthesia for extraction of senile cataract. *Acta Anaesthesiol. Scand.* 1982; **26**: 291–6.

163. Riis J., Lomholt B. Haxholdt O. et al. Immediate and long-term mental recovery from general versus epidural anaesthesia in elderly patients. *Acta Anaesthesiol. Scand.* 1983; **27**: 44–9.

164. Chung F. F., Chung A., Meier R. H., Lautenschlaeger E., Seyone C. Comparison of perioperative mental function after general anaesthesia and spinal anaesthesia with IV sedation. *Can. J. Anaesth.* 1989; **36**: 283–7.

165. Asbjorn J., Jakobsen B. W., Pilegaard H. K. Mental function in elderly men after surgery during epidural anaesthesia. *Acta Anaesthesiol. Scand.* 1989; **33**: 369–73.

166. Jones M. J. T. The influence of anaesthetic methods on mental function. *Acta Chir., Scand.* 1988; Suppl. 550: 169–76.
167. Teasdale C., McCrum A., Williams N. B., Horton R. E. A randomised controlled trial to compare local with general anaesthesia for short-stay inguinal hernia repair. *Ann. R. Coll. Surg. Eng.* 1982; **64**: 238–42.
168. Cullen M. L., Staren E. D., El-Ganzouri, Logas W. G., Inankovich A. D., Economu S. G. Continuous epidural infusion for analgesia after major abdominal operations. A randomised prospective double-blind study. *Surgery* 1985; **98**: 718–28.
169. Valentin N., Lomholt B., Jensen J. S., Hejgaard N., Kreiner S. Spinal or general anaesthesia for surgery of the fractured hip. *Brit. J. Anaesth.* 1986; **58**: 284–91.
170. Kehlet H. Anaesthetic technique and surgical convalescence. *Acta Chir. Scand.* 1988; Supp. 550: 182–91.
171. McInnes C. Cancer ward. *New Society* 1976; **36**: 232.
172. Roizen M. F. Should we all have a sympathectomy at birth? Or at least preoperatively? *Anesthesiology* 1988; **68**: 482–4.
173. Nielsen K. K., Andersen K. Asbjorn J., Vork F., Ohrt-Nissen A. Blood loss in transurethral prostatectomy. Epidural vs. general anaesthesia. *Int. Urol. Nephrol.* 1987; **19**: 287–92.

5

Intrathecal and epidural drug spread

M. S. Brockway,
J. A. W. Wildsmith

Whether a local anaesthetic or an opioid is injected into the spine to produce analgesia after surgery, its effectiveness will depend upon it reaching the appropriate point in the pain pathway. The factors that govern the spread of these drugs within the intrathecal and epidural compartments have considerable practical relevance since the target receptors are located either in the spinal cord or in that portion of the nerve root that lies in the vertebral canal. The first requirement for understanding the mechanisms of such drug spread is a knowledge of the anatomy and physiology of the vertebral canal. It is emphasized that the following discussion applies to the normal spine.

Boundaries of the vertebral canal

The vertebral canal extends from the foramen magnum to the sacral hiatus. It is formed by the dorsal spines, pedicles and laminae (the 'neural arch') of successive vertebrae (7 cervical, 12 thoracic, 5 lumbar, 5 sacral) and the ligaments and discs connecting them. The curves of the vertebral column are mirrored in the canal with primary anterior concave curves in the thoracic and sacral regions and secondary posterior curves in the cervical and lumbar regions.[1] In the supine position the 'high' points of the curves are C5 and L3/4 interspace, whilst the 'low' points are T5 and S2 (Fig. 5.1).[1]

The canal is lined by periosteum, or 'parietal dura', which is continuous with the endosteal layer of cerebral dura mater and forms the outer border of the epidural space. The cross-sectional area of the canal increases from above downwards and is roughly triangular in cross-section (narrow posteriorly and wider anteriorly) although it tends to be more oval in the cervical and circular in the upper thoracic region. The dural sac forms the inner boundary, and determines the cross-sectional shape, of the epidural

111

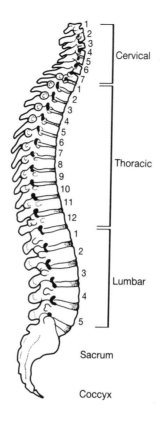

Figure 5.1 Lateral view of the vertebral column.

space. Usually the sac lies in the anterior part of the vertebral canal, dividing the epidural space into a small anterior compartment (roughly 10 per cent of the total) and two larger posterolateral compartments (90 per cent) (Fig. 5.2).

The distance from the posterior border of the canal to the dura varies according to spinal segment. It may be as little as 1 mm in the cervical region and up to 6 mm in the lumbar region, although the space itself is largest in the sacral region because of the absence of the dural sac. In the cervical region the narrowness of the canal means that there is very little epidural space and it is not uncommon for the two layers of dura to be in contact between C1 and C3 so that the space is obliterated altogether. At the foramen magnum the two layers fuse so that further cephalad spread of solution from the epidural space is not possible.

Computerized axial tomography has demonstrated that the dorsal part of the epidural space has a sawtooth pattern[2] such that it is narrowest near the cephalad lamina and widest near the caudad one. This occurs

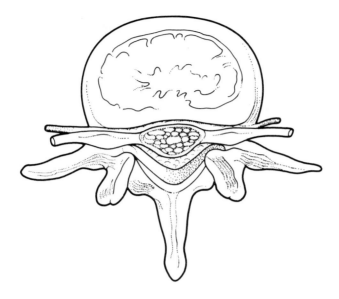

Figure 5.2 Cross-sectional view of a vertebra and the vertebral canal showing the small anterior compartment and larger posterolateral compartments of the epidural space.

because the ligamentum flavum is attached to the anterior aspect of the cephalad lamina and the posterior aspect of the caudad lamina (Fig. 5.3). This suggests that the epidural space should be entered close to the caudad lamina rather than the cephalad lamina. The ventral epidural space also varies in depth, being large behind the vertebral body and smaller behind the protruding intervertebral disc.[3]

There are many openings in the vertebral canal, most notably the 29 pairs of intervertebral foramina, 25 of which face laterally and 4 (sacral)

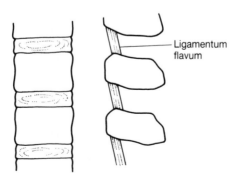

Ligamentum flavum

Figure 5.3 The ligamentum flavum forms a sawtooth posterior border to the epidural space.

anteriorly. Generally they increase in diameter from above downwards, except between C5–T1 and L4–S1 through which larger spinal nerves pass. The vertebral canal communicates with the thoracic and abdominal cavities through these foramina, and also with the cranial cavity through the foramen magnum. The sacrococcygeal ligament usually completely seals the sacral hiatus.

Contents of the vertebral canal

Epidural space

The dorsal and ventral nerve roots cross the epidural space from the dural sac (see later) to the two intervertebral foramina present at each segmental level. The nerves lie in the posterolateral part of the space and become progressively longer and more oblique from above downwards. At the intervertebral foramina the nerves (together with fat and blood vessels) are tethered to the walls by connective tissue known as 'Charpy's ligaments'. It is generally held that with increasing age the foramina offer an increasing barrier, to the point of complete occlusion in some cases,[4, 5] although this is not the case with the anterior sacral foramina.[3, 6]

Epidural fat, which is very vascular and has a semi-fluid consistency, fills the remaining space. The amount was thought to be proportional to body fat,[7] but recent work has demonstrated that this is not so.[8] The nature of the fat changes with age, such that it offers increasing resistance to injection.[7] The epidural veins (the plexus of Batson) are large, valveless and lie mainly in the anterolateral part of the space. They have numerous connections at all segmental levels, including the sacral (and hence iliac and uterine) venous plexus, and the abdominal and thoracic veins. Thus pressure changes within these body cavities are reflected in the epidural veins, most notably in pregnancy when the veins are distended and the effective volume of the epidural space decreased (see later). Lymphatics and arteries, which are relatively small, pass through the intervertebral foramina.

In 1986 Blomberg,[8] using a technique he devised and called epiduroscopy, reported the existence in cadavers of dorsal midline strands connecting the dura mater to the ligamentum flavum. These were seen to cause a fold in the dura mater – the plica mediana dorsalis. The existence of such connective structures had been suggested by Luyendijk in 1963 when he observed a midline defect during peridurography.[3] He assumed that this fold was caused by median attachment to the vertebral laminae, but until Blomberg's study the evidence had been circumstantial. The strands were seen to narrow the epidural space in the midline, an observation which contrasts with the popular belief that the space is widest at this point. Indeed Blomberg punctured the dura mater on four occasions where heavy dorsomedian connections had closely attached it to the ligamentum flavum. The strands were particularly well developed in the region of the vertebral arches and were seen to be responsible for altering catheter direction by as much as 180 degrees, especially as the amount of catheter in the space increased. In two cases the strands formed a complete membrane which prevented the catheter crossing from one side to the other.

Savolaine and colleagues[9] using computerized tomography confirmed the midline division of the posterior epidural space. In addition they demonstrated connective tissue bands that appeared to originate from the plica mediana dorsalis and extend laterally, thus effectively subdividing the posterolateral compartments of the epidural space into anterior and posterior sections (Fig. 5.4). The same investigators were also able to demonstrate these structures during dissection of cadavers, thus eliminating the possibility that they were artifactual.

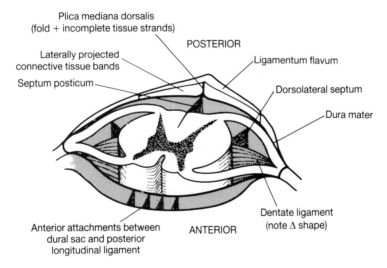

Figure 5.4 Cross-section of the vertebral canal showing the ligaments and connective tissue of the epidural and intrathecal spaces.

The posterior longitudinal ligament which runs down the posterior aspect of the vertebral bodies and discs, has numerous connections to the anterior dural sac. The close attachment or even opposition of the dural sac to the anterior canal wall may serve to separate the ventral compartment and therefore prevent the entry of fluid from the dorsal parts of the epidural space. These dorsal compartments of the space are preferentially filled when contrast[9] or resin is injected,[10] probably because injected fluid follows the path of least resistance. Injected contrast medium is frequently seen to run through the intervertebral foramina into the paravertebral space, so confirming the direct connection between them.[9, 11]

The dural sac

The inner layer of dura mater in the vertebral canal is continuous with the meningeal layer in the cranial cavity. It is composed of dense longitudinal fibres and forms the dural sac. The dura is firmly attached to, and extends caudally from, the foramen magnum. The sac usually terminates at the lower border of the second sacral segment (lower in children) where it is pierced by the filum terminale (a continuation of the pia mater) which runs caudally (closely invested by dura) to attach to periosteum on the posterior surface of the coccyx. The filum teminale serves to stabilize both the dural sac and the spinal cord. The sac is further stabilized by the spinal nerves, fibrous connections to the posterior longitudinal ligament anteriorly (especially inferiorly) and to the ligamentum flavum posteriorly (see earlier). These attachments are probably responsible for the roughly triangular cross sectional shape (apex posteriorly) of the dural sac.[3]

The arachnoid mater is closely applied to the inner surface of the dura mater, but there is a potential space, the subdural space, between them. Extensions of the arachnoid and dura mater continue along the spinal nerves, progressively thinning to become continuous with the coverings of the peripheral nerves. Initially each of the dural 'cuffs' so formed contains a pocket of cerebrospinal fluid (CSF). In addition, the dura is pierced at these points by the numerous veins, arteries and lymphatics which pass between the subarachnoid and the epidural spaces. Arachnoid granulations protrude through the dural cuffs and communicate with the epidural veins and lymphatics. This facilitates drainage of CSF and the removal of foreign material. It is not difficult to understand that this region may also allow the rapid transfer of drugs from the epidural space to the CSF.

The subarachnoid space lies deep to the arachnoid mater. It contains CSF, numerous delicate trabeculations running between the arachnoid and pia maters, the spinal cord and the dorsal and ventral nerve roots. The spinal cord extends from the medulla oblongata, with which it is continuous, and ends as the conus medullaris at the lower border of the first lumbar vertebra (the exact level is variable, and is closer to L3 in the neonate). It has an average length of 45 cm and weight of 30 g in the adult male. The cord is elliptical in cross-section (greater transverse diameter at all levels) and tapers caudally except for two distinct expansions. The first, and larger of these, is the cervicothoracic enlargement. It commences a little below the foramen magnum, reaches maximum width at the level of C5, tapers off at T2, and reflects the extensive innervation of the upper limb. The second, the lumbosacral enlargement (innervating the lower limbs), is situated between the ninth and twelfth thoracic vertebrae. The cord and the nerve roots are closely covered by a delicate membrane known as the pia mater. The blood vessels supplying the cord lie within this tissue.

There are 31 pairs of spinal nerves (8 cervical, 12 thoracic, 5 lumbar, 5 sacral and 1 coccygeal) and each nerve has a dorsal and a ventral root. The roots are in fact formed from several smaller rootlets or fibrils and every dorsal root has a ganglion. The increasing obliquity of the nerve roots means that the lumbar and sacral roots lie freely in the CSF below the level of the conus medullaris (i.e. below the lower border of L1) and form the cauda equina. The subarachnoid space extends separately along each nerve root as far as the dorsal root ganglion, thereafter the arachnoid and pia mater merge and continue as the perineural tissue of the spinal nerves.

Within the CSF several connective tissue strands or trabeculae are found. The pattern of these varies considerably between individuals, but there are generally far more trabeculae along the dorsal aspect of the cord than ventrally (Fig. 5.4).[12] In most subjects a midline dorsal septum, the 'septum posticum'[12, 14] extends typically from the midcervical to lumbar regions. This septum usually has irregular perforations and tends to be increasingly fenestrated towards its upper and lower ends. It is generally attached to the pia mater along the course of the dorsal vein of the spinal cord.[12] Anatomical studies have suggested that the septum tends to thicken with increasing age.[13]

Lateral to the septum posticum two dorsolateral septae extend from the region of the dorsal rootlets and attach them to the dorsolateral arachnoid mater. They tend to be more irregular and fenestrated than the septum posticum and generally extend further rostrally and caudally, probably serving to tether the dorsal rootlets and keep them clear of the lateral parts of the spinal cord.[12] Unlike the septum posticum these trabeculations tend to atrophy with age.[13] Further lateral projections from the pia, known as denticulate or dentate ligaments, which are more substantial then the other trabeculations,[13] attach to the dura mater and act to support the spinal cord. There are no attachments anterior to the dentate ligaments.

Physiology of the vertebral canal

Epidural Pressure

The presence of a subatmospheric pressure in the epidural space was first reported by Janzen in 1926[15] and Gutierrez described the hanging drop sign in 1932.[16] In the thoracic region the pressure is due largely to transmission of the negative intrathoracic pressure through the intervertebral foramina.

It may be as low as -10 cm H_2O,[11] especially on deep inspiration.[17] The lowest pressures are recorded in the upper and middle thoracic regions and increases with distance from the thorax so that they are least negative (if negative at all) in the lumbar and sacral regions.[11, 18] The negative pressure in the thoracic and cervical regions is enhanced when sitting and when the spine is flexed,[19] whereas in chronic obstructive airways disease, it may cease to be negative. Coughing and the valsalva manoeuvres have been shown to increase the epidural pressure in all regions.[11, 18]

During lumbar epidural blockade the predominant cause of the negative pressure is indentation of the dura mater by the needle (especially if it is a blunt one). It is evident therefore that negative pressure is a poor sign for the recognition of entry into the lumbar epidural space. The negative pressure increases as the needle is advanced[7] and one investigator[20] obtained a pressure of -14 cm H_2O when indenting the dura with a blunt needle. Usubiaga recorded figures of -21 cm H_2O just prior to dural puncture.[11]

Usubiaga and his colleagues have observed cyclical variations in epidural pressure.[18] Firstly, small pressure waves, synchronous with arterial pulsation, were seen in all the thoracic and cervical recordings (5 of each), in 3 of the 6 lumbar traces, but never in the (4) sacral recordings. Larger amplitude variations, synchronous with respiration, were noted in 13 out of 15 patients. In the cervical and thoracic regions the pressure increased with expiration and decreased with inspiration, whereas in the lumbar region (unlike CSF, discussed later) the reverse was noted. These patterns were also found in the superior and inferior venae cavae respectively. When the pressure in each venous system was elevated independently (Queckenstedt manoeuvre or abdominal compression), the epidural pressure change was largely confined to the adjoining space. A valsalva manoeuvre or cough resulted in increased epidural pressure except in the sacral region.

From these observations it was concluded that the epidural space has three functional compartments: the cervico-thoracic, which is the largest, and influenced by pressure changes in the superior venae cava; the lumbar, which is influenced by intra-abdominal pressure; and finally the sacral canal, which has no negative pressure, no pressure oscillations and does not respond to abdominal compression. It is thought that the lipid tissue of the epidural space serves to isolate the regions allowing them to reflect the pressure changes in the cavities with which they communicate most directly.

Factors affecting epidural drug spread

Many controlled clinical studies have closely examined the spread of fluid injected into the epidural (and subarachnoid) spaces. The most objective indicator of this spread is the extent of local anaesthetic block, although it must be recognized that some of the drug will have spread more widely than is apparent, but not in a concentration sufficient to cause neural blockade. Such studies have indicated the important factors which influence spread and this information may be applied to other classes of drug, although the precise influences on their spread may be different.

With regard to epidural spread the many factors involved have been reviewed extensively by Park,[21] and their variable interactions would appear to be the cause of the unpredictability associated with this block.

Anatomical variation

Despite the subdivision of the epidural space by the connective tissue bands described earlier, blockade is usually bilateral and complete. This implies that these bands do not constitute a significant barrier to spread, although unilateral blocks have been reported,[22, 23] and it is conceivable that occasionally these structures may be responsible. As stated earlier, Blomberg was able to observe the plica mediana dorsalis impeding catheter insertion,[8] and difficulty filling both sides of the epidural space have been attributed to this.[24] Nevertheless the full implication of the plica and other epidural structures remains to be evaluated.

The narrower, or possibly even obliterated, cervical epidural space has been implicated in the restriction of the spread of local anaesthetic within the region[19] and the consequent rarity of cervical nerve blockade in the presence of dense thoracic block. The smaller volume of the spinal canal and the larger size of the dural sac in the upper parts of the spine mean that less volume is required to fill the space than in the lumbar region. Conversely injection of a given amount of local anaesthetic often produces more extensive blockade in the cervical and upper thoracic regions than in the lumbar region.[21] Furthermore, it is possible that greater leakage of solution will occur through the larger intervertebral foramina present in the lower regions of the spine.

It has been suggested that the smaller volume of the upper parts of the epidural space combined with the greater negative pressure are the reasons for greater cephalad spread than caudad spread, seen after lumbar epidural injection.[21] The greater size of some nerve roots (e.g. L5, S1 and the roots of the brachial plexus) is responsible for slow onset of block within their distribution.[7]

Epidural pressure

The effect of the injection of fluid into the epidural space on epidural pressure has been studied closely.[11] The initial injection follows the path of least resistance, usually to those areas where the pressure is most negative. As the pressure becomes positive the solution begins to leak from the space[25, 26] or displace other fluids from the vertebral canal.[27]

Usubiaga reported that injection caused epidural pressure to increase by as much as 60 cm H_2O,[11, 18] but it has been suggested that the extent of the pressure rise is limited by displacement of the CSF.[28] This theory is supported by the observation that rapid injection in particular can increase intracranial pressure.[7, 27] The greatest pressure changes are seen with lumbar injection in the sitting position, and the lowest with sacral injection. After the initial increase the pressure falls exponentially towards the original baseline over a ten minute period, with most of the decrease occurring in the first two minutes, especially in younger patients.

Usubiaga[11] recorded epidural pressure at spaces adjacent to the injection site and showed delayed and somewhat less marked increases up to 4 segments away, but at more distant sites the pressure traces were unaltered. The residual epidural pressure (persisting after the initial steep decline) is greater in older patients, indicating decreased epidural space compliance.[11] The reasons for this may include less passage of fluid through the intervertebral foramina and the decreased compliance of epidural fat seen with advancing years.

When residual pressure was plotted against block height it was noted that, in general, the higher the pressure then the greater the spread (after ten minutes).[11] This, and a similar finding in a separate study,[29] suggested that if the normal epidural pressure was artificially increased then a solution could be made to spread further. However, other authors have not been able to demonstrate any relationship between residual pressure and spread.[28, 30] Certainly the pressure immediately after injection appears to be unrelated to the subsequent block height.[26]

Age/segmental dose requirement

In 1969 Bromage introduced the concept of a segmental dose requirement (SDR), which he defined as the mass of drug required to block a segment.[31] He found that this was greatest (1.5 ml) at 19 years of age and that it decreased linearly thereafter. Sharrock and colleagues reported a SDR of 1.3 ml up to 40 years of age, but while agreeing on the decreased volume required in the elderly they were unable to demonstrate a linear relationship[32] and several other workers have also disputed this.[26, 33–5]

Since the volume of the epidural space varies from region to region it is unlikely that the volume required to block each segment will be the same. Furthermore the SDR has been shown to increase with the total dose administered.[26, 34] Park[26] demonstrated that the SDR was 0.67 ml when 10 ml of lignocaine were injected, but that it increased to 1.11 ml with a 20 ml injection. Grundy[34] reported a similar response with bupivacaine, doubling the volume from 10 to 20 ml blocked only three additional segments (from 16.9 to 19.7).

Although the view that less solution escapes through the intervertebral foramina in the elderly is widely held to cause greater spread, Luyendijk found no strong evidence to support this; however, he did admit to an impression of some decrease in permeability.[3] Further explanations for the greater effect of epidural local anaesthetics in the elderly could be the altered contours and decreased numbers of myelinated nerves that occur with age. In addition the connective tissue that envelops the nerves becomes thinner with the generalized deterioration of mucopolysacharides that occurs with ageing. This would allow greater penetration by the local anaesthetic agents. Another aspect of ageing that has been implicated in enhancement of local anaesthetic activity is that of atherosclerosis. Bromage found that SDR was decreased in such patients,[36] but as explained earlier the SDR varies with the dose administered.

Height

Tall patients are said to require larger doses of local anaesthetic to block a given number of segments, but the correlation with height is poor.[19] This is not surprising since the length of the spine is not as variable as height in the adult population.

Weight

Generally obese patients carry most of their excess fat subcutaneously, but they also tend to have increased deposits in all other areas where fat occurs.[7, 19] However Blomberg could find no correlation between the amount of epidural and subcutaneous fat,[8] and his observation is borne out by the findings of Duggan and colleagues[33] who were unable to demonstrate any relation between weight and block height. Further investigation is required.

Posture

The use of gravity and positioning are of limited value in predicting the spread of epidural blockade, possibly because of the influences of pressure, but may be of some clinical use. Usubiaga[11] demonstrated preferential lateral spread to the paravertbral space, although it should be noted that the spread of contrast agents (which have relatively high specific gravities) may be different from that of local anaesthetics. Other authors have reported marginally earlier onset and a slight increase in extent and duration of blockade on the dependent side[37, 38] whilst repositioning during continuous epidural infusion has resulted in changes in the pattern of blockade.[39]

When local anaesthetic is deliverd by continuous infusion the mechanism of spread is somewhat different from that of bolus injection. With a bolus the high injection pressure results in a jet, or jets, from the catheter (or needle), and this pressure is responsible for spread of solution away from the tip. With an infusion technique the solution emerges from the catheter at low pressure, spread is facilitated by the use of large volumes and increasing flow rates.[19] To increase the extent or density of blockade with an infusion technique would take a considerable amount of time because of the slow spread from the catheter, therefore it is usual practice to use a supplemental bolus. Gravity exerts more influence on epidural infusions than it does for bolus injections; Schweitzer has shown that with bolus injection there is approximately twice as much spread up the spine compared to down, but that with infusions the ratio is decreased to 4:3 with 20 ml.h^{-1} and reversed to 1:2 with 10 ml.h^{-1}.[19]

Injection technique

Rate of injection would appear to have little effect on subsequent blockade. Grundy and colleagues[34] reported an increase in block height of less than one segment with a threefold variation of rate of injection and other investigators have reported similar findings.[30, 40] Despite this small increase in mean spread, rapid injection is also associated with an increased incidence of incomplete block and of patient discomfort.[40] A possible associated decrease in duration may be due to each nerve being exposed to a smaller amount of drug.[21] Cephalad *orientation of needle bevel* resulted in a 1–2 segment increase in cephalad spread compared to caudal spread, in patients over 40 years of age, whereas in a younger population no effect was seen.[41]

The extent of sensory blockade is often said to be related to the *volume and dose* injected, but the nature of the relationship is not straightforward and has led to the view that 'the height of analgesia produced by a given volume of solution is one of the great uncertainties of anaesthesia'.[4] A recent study found virtually identical extent of blockade irrespective of the dose, volume or concentration of the solution injected, so contradicting the opening premise of this paragraph.[33] Furthermore, a smaller range of spread and more symmetrical blocks with the lower volumes was noted, prompting the conclusion that perhaps more predictable epidural block would follow the injection of a low volume of concentrated solution. Other studies[26, 34] found that increases in volume and dose did increase spread, but that the difference were slight. It is more appropriate to match the *site of injection* to the level of segmental blockade required, rather than attempting to extend the block with increasing amounts of local anaesthetic. Furthermore, the onset of blockade in the most relevant dermatomes will be quicker. This, of course, is not a new idea because Dogliotti's original description of epidural blockade emphasized the ability to match the distribution of blockade to that of surgery as the main advantage of the procedure over intrathecal block.[42]

Local anaesthetic solution will follow a path of least resistance when injected rather than filling the epidural space in an even manner, and drug is absorbed rapidly into the tissues, or the solution may escape through the intervertebral foramina. This effect may be exaggerated when an incremental technique is employed, for the path probably tends to be repeatedly followed and the drug absorbed into the same tissue or escape using the same exit. This may explain the relatively small effects that volume and dose appear to exert on the extent of blockade, and the occasional patchy block which is observed when an incremental technique is employed. A continuous injection has been recommended to avoid this effect.[43] Duggan and colleagues[33] used a 'single injection through needle' technique and reported a complete absence of incomplete or unilateral blocks. Other investigators comparing continuous and incremental injection have reported[44] none or only slight benefit from continuous injection.[21]

Routes of escape

Theoretically there are several ways that a solution may escape from the epidural space:

1.   passage through the intervertebral foramina;
2.   absorption of drug into the circulation which occurs immediately after injection and increases with increasing concentration of drug;[45, 46] the addition of adrenaline may decrease this absorption especially with lignocaine;
3.   diffusion into the neural and other tissues (which is further increased if using carbonated or alkalinized solutions);
4.   passage along the needle whilst it remains *in situ* (i.e. drip back) and possibly along the track after its removal. It is conceivable that escape may be promoted by increased epidural pressure, and Usubiaga has reported increased leak back along the needle in subjects with higher residual pressures.[11]

Pregnancy

Pregnancy merits special consideration firstly because of the physiological changes which occur and their effect on the epidural space, and secondly because of the large number of blocks performed in obstetrics. There is an increase in intra-abdominal pressure, and venous engorgement of the epidural space (especially during uterine contractions) resulting in a predictable increase in baseline epidural pressure. Usubiaga and colleagues failed to demonstrate negative pressure in the epidural space of any patients presenting for Caesarean section.[11] The pressure increase is more marked when supine, and during the second stage of labour it may be as high as 10 cm H_2O.[47] Considering the effects of pressure on blockade (see earlier) one might expect greater spread if injection occurred at a time of high pressure (e.g. a contraction) compared to low pressure, but Sivakumaran failed to demonstrate any great difference.[48]

The greater effect of epidural local anaesthetic drugs in pregnancy is unlikely to be the result of a single factor. Engorgement of the veins passing though the intervetrebral foramina will act to impair passage of fluid to the paravertebral space, and a probable hormone-mediated increase in the permeability of the nerve root coverings during pregnancy which permits increased local anaesthetic penetration of the nerve roots.[21] It is implicit therefore that a given amount of local anaesthetic solution will spread further in the longitudinal axis, and will have enhanced performance. However, with appropriate positioning of the patient, engorgement of the epidural veins may be reduced and the influence on the spread of epidural local anaesthetic may be decreased.

Physiology of cerebrospinal fluid

CFS is a clear fluid, with a specific gravity of roughly 1.005 at 37°C (this may be increased slightly in conditions such as old age, uraemia, hypergly-caemia and hypothermia). Its function is to support and protect the brain and spinal cord. It has a hydrogen ion concentration of 40–45 nmol.1^{-1}, is isotonic with plasma (280–290 mosmol.1^{-1}) and has a similar ionic profile (Table 5.1). It contains only trace amounts of protein (hence the total calcium concentration is lower), with the concentration being lowest in the ventricles and greatest in the lumbar region. Small numbers of blood cells are present in healthy CSF.

Table 5.1 Constituents of CSF and plasma

Constituent	CSF	Plasma
Na$^+$ mmol.1^{-1}	140	142
Cl$^-$ mmol.1^{-1}	115	98
K$^+$ mmol.1^{-1}	2.9	4.5
Urea mmol.1^{-1}	5.0	5.0
Glocose mmol.1^{-1}	4.5	5.0
HCO$_3$_ mmol.1^{-1}	22	25
Ca^{2+} mmol.1^{-1}	1.2	2.3
Mg^{2+} mmol.1^{-1}	1.0	0.8
Protein mg.dl^{-1}	20–40	6000–8000

The difference between CSF and plasma imply that it is actively secreted rather than an ultrafiltrate. This is confirmed by the effects of drugs that influence sodium transport (such as acetazolamide) have on CSF composition and rate of formation. It is formed by the choroid plexi which lie in the ependyma of the walls of the lateral and fourth ventricles. The total volume of CSF in the adult is approximately 130 ml and the average daily production 150 ml, although this may increase up to three-fold should the volume be low, and decrease when pressure is raised. CSF formation also varies linearly with serum osmolality, reducing when this is increased and vice versa.

From the lateral ventricles CSF passes to the third and then the fourth ventricle through the interventricular foramina of Munro and the aqueduct of Sylvius. It reaches the cisterna magna and the cerebral subarachnoid space through the foramina of Luschka and Magendie. Most flows upwards over the brain and is reabsorbed through the arachnoid villi into the superior sagittal and transverse sinuses (and the other sinuses to a lesser extent). Spinal CSF accounts for about 35 ml of the total. The majority is in the area of the cauda equina and some may drain into local venous plexi through small valves,[49] but most returns to the cranial cavity.

There is no active CSF flow within the vertebral canal, the character of the fluid being maintained by a combination of diffusion and alterations in posture. The normal CSF pressure in the lumbar region is 60–100 mm H_2O in the lateral position and 200–250 mm H_2O when sitting. The pressure oscillates in time with both arterial pulsation and respiration. Respiration can cause pressure changes of up to 30 mm H_2O (an increase with expiration, a decrease with inspiration), whilst the arterial waves may have an amplitude of 2–15 mm H_2O.[18] These pressure variations are consistent throughout the CSF unlike the situation in the epidural space (see earlier).

Factors affecting intrathecal spread of drug

The most important determinants of spread of solution through the CSF have been reviewed by Greene[50] and may be summarized as follows:

Solution baricity. Using 0.5% amethocaine, Brown and his colleagues[51] found that baricity had a major effect on the spread of analgesia. The solution was injected at the third lumbar interspace in patients placed in the lateral horizontal position and turned supine immediately afterwards. The hyperbaric solution resulted in a mean block to T5 and and isobaric to T10. The hypobaric solution gave a mean level of T11, but the blocks were patchy and of poor quality. Increasing the dose injected from 10 to 15 mg had no effect on the level of spread achieved with any solution, but did increase duration.

Patient posture.   Posture has been used since the time of Barker's[1] classical descriptions to aid or restrict spread of injected solution. If a patient is turned supine immediately after injection at the third or fourth lumbar interspace, the solution will be at the apex of the lumbar spinal curve. Gravity will thus cause a hyperbaric solution to spread down from the apex in both sacral and thoracic directions. With a hyperbaric solution it is not necessary to use the Trendelenberg position to ensure spread to mid-thoracic level. Sinclair and colleagues[52] found that this manoeuvre increased the variability of height of block and increased the incidence of blocks extending into the cervical region. Accentuation of the lumbar curve in pregnancy may explain in part the increased spread seen when spinal anaesthesia is performed with a hyperbaric solution for Caesarean section. Conversely, flexion of the hips in the supine position reduces the lumbar curve and has been shown to reduce the spread of hyperbaric solutions.[53]

A major reason for using posture to control the spread of hyperbaric solutions is to try to restrict spread to the lower limbs and perineum. Wildsmith and colleagues[54] investigated the effect of maintaining both the lateral and sitting positions for 5 minutes after the injection of hyperbaric or isobaric solutions of amethocaine. They concluded that if posture is to be used to control the spread of a hyperbaric solution, then the posture must be maintained for considerably longer (>5 mins) than is often practised. They also found that posture had no effect at all on the spread of a truly isobaric solution, which they recommended for producing a block restricted to the legs or perineum.

Volume and rate of injection.   Increasing the volume of a spinal anesthetic injection usually increases the dose of drug injected. McClure and colleagues devised a study in which a standard dose of amethocaine was dissolved in 1, 2 or 4 ml of isobaric solution.[55] There was very little difference in mean spread with the different volumes, but the larger the volume injected, the greater was the range of blocks – i.e. predictability was reduced. Slowing the rate of injection of 4 ml reduced the range of blocks produced and made the solution more predictable. It was concluded that the most predictable spinal blocks would be produced by injecting a low volume solution at a slow rate.

Level of injection.   It is probable that the level of injection will have some effect on the ultimate height of block. With plain solutions of bupivacaine which is slightly hypobaric increase in the level of injection by only one interspace has been shown to produce a significantly higher level of block.[56] Much the same effect will usually be seen with a hyperbaric solution, but rather unusual blocks are sometimes seen with such preparations if they are injected at levels other than the third lumbar interspace. When injected at that level, a hyperbaric solution will, in the supine patient, spread with gravity in both caudad and cephalad directions. However, with a lower or higher injection (or in a patient with an abnormal lordosis) the solution may only spread in either a caudad *or* a cephalad direction.

Patient characteristics.   Many anaesthetists relate the dose of local anaesthetic that they use in a spinal anaesthetic to the patient's height or weight. While restricted spread is sometimes seen in the very thin patient, and the opposite in the obese, many studies have found that spread correlates very poorly with patient size, certainly within the adult range. McCulloch and Littlewood[57] have shown that there is some increase in spread in the obese patient, but the range of blocks is so wide that height, weight and lean body mass are of very little predictive help. Similarly, some correlation has been shown between patient age and intrathecal spread,[58, 59] but again the range of blocks seen in any particular age group is too wide for the information to be of any practical help.

Effect of clinical interactions.   The results of the studies outlined have indicated how the major factors affect the spread of local anesthetic solution after intrathecal injection. However, it is important to appreciate that these studies were performed in healthy patients under very carefully controlled conditions. In the routine clinical situation variations in technique, differences in solution composition, and individual patient factors (e.g. distortion of the spine with age) may individually or together result in more variable spread.

For instance, Axelsson and colleagues[60] studied the spread of plain bupivacaine 0.5% in patients who were sitting for 2 minutes after injection and then placed in the lithotomy position. They found that cephalad spread was proportional to the logarithm of the volume injected. However Chambers and his colleagues[61] found that volume had no effect on the spread of hyperbaric 0.5% bupivacaine, but that there was an effect on the spread of hyperbaric 0.75% bupivacaine. Others[61, 62] have in fact demonstrated some relationship between volume injected and the spread of hyperbaric 0.5% bupivacaine.

Such contradictory results may be due to a number of factors, including simple chance. It is important to remember that any technique of spinal anesthesia results in a range of blocks, even when it is applied consistently by a single practitioner. Therefore it is not surprising that there should be some variation between the results of studies in which there may be subtle, seemingly irrelevant variations in technique, drug composition and patient characteristics. Too many investigators have not appreciated the importance of keeping every factor completely constant except the one being studied.

Currently epidurals would appear to offer greater scope in the management of postoperative pain than spinal injection. The reasons for this are twofold; firstly, the use of a catheter for prolonged drug administration (although the recent advent of spinal catheters may obviate this aspect) and secondly, by appropriate positioning of the catheter, the ability to provide selective blockade.

References

1. Barker A. E. A report on clinical experiences with spinal analgesia in 100 cases, and some reflections on the procedure. *Brit. Med. J.*. 1907; **1**: 665–74.
2. Reynolds A. F. Jr., Roberts P. A., Pollay M., Stratemeier P. H. Quantitative anatomy of the thoracolumbar epidural space. *Neurosurgery*. 1985; **17**: 905–7.
3. Luyendijk W. Canalography. *J. Belge Radiol*. 1963; **46**: 236–54.
4. Atkinson R. S., Rushman G. B., Lee J. A. Spinal analgesia: Intradural; epidural. In: *A Synopsis of Anaesthesia, 10th edition*. Bristol: Wright, 1987: 662–721.
5. Reynolds F. J. M. Spinal and epidural block. In: Churchill Davidson H. C. *A Practice of Anaesthesia, 5th edition*. London: Lloyd-Luke, 1984: 856–92.
6. Luyendijk W., Van Voorthuisen A. E. Contrast examination of the spinal epidural space. *Acta Scand. Radiol*. 1966; **5**: 1051–66.
7. Cousins M. J., Bromage P. R. Epidural neural blockade. In: Cousins M. J., Bridenbaugh P. O. *Neural Blockade in Clinical Anesthesia and Management of Pain, 2nd edition*. Philadelphia: Lippincott, 1988: 253–360.
8. Blomberg R. The dorsomedian connective tissue band in the lumbar epidural space of humans: an anatomical study using epiduroscopy in autopsy cases. *Anesthesia and Analgesia*. 1986; **65**: 747–52.
9. Savolaine E. R., Pandaya J. B., Greenblatt S. H., Conover S. R. Anatomy of the human lumbar epidural space: new insights using CT-Epidurography. *Anesthseiol*. 1988; **68**: 217–20.
10. Harrison G. R., Parkin I. G., Shah J. L. Resin injection of the lumbar extradural space. *Brit. J. Anaesth*. 1985; **57**: 333–6.
11. Usubiaga J. E., Wikinski J. A., Usubiaga L. E. Epidural pressure and its relation to spread of anesthetic solutions in the epidural space. *Anesthesia and analgesia*. 1967; **46**: 440–6.
12. Nauta H. J. E., Dolan E., Yasargil M. G. Microsurgical anatomy of the spinal subarachnoid space. *Surg. Neurol*. 1983; **19**: 431–7.
13. Key E. A. H., Retzius M. G. *Studien in der Nerven-systems und des Bindegewebs*. Stockholm: Samson and Wallin, 1879.
14. Di Chiro G., Timins E. L. Spinal myelography and the septum posticum. *Radiol*. 1974; **111**: 319–27.
15. Janzen E. Der negative vorschlag bei lumbalpunktion. *Deutsche Z Nerven Heilk*. 1926; **94**: 280–92.
16. Gutierrez A. Valor de la aspiracion liquida en el espacio peridural en la anestesia preidural. *Rev. Circulation, Buenos Aires*. 1933; **12**: 225.
17. Bryce-Smith R. Pressures in the extra-dural space. *Anaesthesia*. 1950; **5**: 213–6.
18. Usubiaga J. E., Moya F., Usubiaga L. E. Effect of thoracic and abdominal

pressure changes on the epidural space pressure. *Brit. J. Anaesthesia.* 1967; **39**: 612–8.

19. Armitage E. N. Lumbar and thoracic epidural anaesthesia. In: Wildsmith J. A. W., Armitage E. N. *Principles and Practice of Regional Anaesthesia.* Edinburgh: Churchill Livingston, 1987; 81–102.

20. Eaton L. M., Observations on the negative pressure in the epidural space. *Mayo Clin. Proc.* 1939; **14**: 566.

21. Park W. Y. Factors influencing the distribution of local anesthetics in the epidural space. *Reg. Anesthesia.* 1988; **13**: 49–57.

22. Ducrow N. The occurrence of unblocked segments during continuous lumbar epidural analgesia for pain relief in labour. *Brit. J. Anaesthesia.* 1971; **43**: 1172–3.

23. Caseby N. G. Epidural analgesia for the surgical induction of labour. *Brit. J. Anaesthesia.* 1974; **46**: 747–51.

24. Robertson G. H., Hatten H. P., Hesselink J. H. Epidurography: selective catheter technique and review of 53 cases. *Amer. J. Radiol.* 1979; **132**: 787–93.

25. Dogliotti A. M. A new method of block anaesthesia. Segmental peridural spinal anesthesia. *Amer. J. Surg.* 1933; **20**: 107–18.

26. Park W. Y., Hagins F. M., Rivat E. L., Macnamara T. E. Age and epidural dose response in adult men. *Anesthesiol.* 1982; **56**: 318–20.

27. Wildsmith J. A. W. Extradural blockade and intracranial pressure. *Brit. J. Anaesthesia.* 1986; **58**: 579.

28. Paul D. L., Wildsmith J. A. W. Extradural pressure following the injection of two volumes of bupivacaine. *Brit. J. Anaesthesia.* 1989; **62**: 368–72.

29. Nishimura N., Kitahara T., Kusakafe T. The spread of lidocaine and I[131] solution in the epidural space. *Anesthesiol.* 1959; **20**: 785–8.

30. Husemeyer R. P., White D. C. Lumbar extradural injection pressures in pregnant women: an investigation of relationships between rate of injection, injection pressures and extent of analgesia. *Brit. J. Anaesthesia.* 1980; **52**: 55–60.

31. Bromage P. R. Ageing and epidural dose requirements. *Brit. J. Anaesthesia.* 1969; **41**: 1016–22.

32. Sharrock N. E. Epidural anesthetic dose responses in patients 20 to 80 years old. *Anesthesiol.* 1978; **49**: 425–8.

33. Duggan J., Bowler G. M. R., McClure J. H., Wildsmith J. A. W. Extradural block with bupivacaine: Influence of dose, volume, concentration and patient characteristics. *Brit. J. Anaesthesia.* 1988; **61**: 324–31.

34. Grundy E. M., Ramamurthy S., Patel K. P., Mani M., Winnie A. P. Epidural analgesia revisited: a statistical study. *Brit. J. Anaesthesia.*

35. Veering B. T., Burm A. G. L., Van Kleef J. W., Hennis P. J. Epidural anaesthesia with bupivacaine: effects of age on neural blockade and pharmacokinetics. *Eur. Soc. Reg. Anaesthesia, 5th Congress Abstracts.* 1986; 36.

36. Bromage P. R. Exaggerated spread of epidural analgesia in arteriosclerotic patients. *Brit. Med. J.* 1962; 1634–8.

37. Apostolou G. A., Zarmakoupis P. K., Mastrokostopoulos G. T. Spread of epidural anesthesia and the lateral position. *Anesthesia and Analgesia.* 1981; **60**: 584–586.

38.   Grundy E. M., Rao L. N., Winnie A. P. Epidural anesthesia and the lateral position. *Anesthesia and Analgesia.* 1978; **57**: 95–97.
39.   Brockway M. S., Noble D., Tunstall M. E. A comparison of 0.08% and 0.0625% bupivacaine for continuous epidural analgesia in labour. *Eur. J. of Anaesthesia.* 1990; **7**: 227–234.
40.   Erdemir H. A., Sopper L. E., Sweet R. B. Studies of factors affecting peridural anesthesia. *Anesthesia and Analgesia.* 1965; **44**: 400–4.
41.   Park W. Y., Poon K. C., Massengale M. D., MacNamara T. E. Direction of needle bevel and epidural anesthetic spread. *Anesthesiol.* 1982; **57**: 327–8.
42.   Dogliotti A. M. Un promettente metodo di anestesia tronculare in studio: La ranchianestesia peridurale segmentaria. *Bull. Mem. Soc. Piemontese Chir.* 1931; **1**: 385–99.
43.   Burn J. M. B., Guyer P. B., Langdon L. The spread of solutions injected into the epidural space; a study using epidurograms in patients with the lumbo-sciatic syndrome. *Brit. J. Aneasthesia.* 1973; **45**: 338–44.
44.   Batra M. S., Bridenbaugh l. D., Levy S. Epidural anesthesia for caesarean section; comparison of bolus and fractionated injection. *Reg. Anesthesia.* 1985; **10**: 50 (A).
45.   Braid D. P., Scott D. B. The systemic absorption of local analgesic drugs. *Brit. J. Anaesthesia.* 1965; **37**: 394–404.
46.   Braid D. P., Scott D. B. Dosage of lignocaine in epidural block in relation to toxicity. *Brit. J. Anaesthesia.* 1966; **38**: 596–602.
47.   Galbert M. W., Marx G. F. Extradural pressures in the parturient patient. *Anesthesiol.* 1974; **40**: 499–502.
48.   Sivakumaran C., Ramanathan S., Chalon J., Satyanarayana T., Turndorf H. Spread of epidural anesthetics and uterine contractions. *Anesthesia and Analgesia.* 1981; **60**: 277–8.
49.   Williams P. L., Warwick R., Dyson M., Bannister L. H. Neurology. In: Williams P. L., Warwick R., Dyson M., Bannister L. H. *Grays Anatomy 37th edition.* Edinburgh: Churchill Livingston, 1989: 859–1243.
50.   Greene N. M. Distribution of local anaesthetic solutions within the subarachnoid space. *Anesthesia and Analgesia.* 1985; **63**: 715–30.
51.   Brown D. T., Wildsmith J. A. W., Covino B. G., Scott D. B. Effect of baracity on spinal anaesthesia with amethocaine. *Brit. J. Anaesthesia.* 1980; **52**: 589–96.
52.   Sinclair C. J., Scott D. B., Edstrom H. H. Effect of the trendelenberg position of spinal anaesthesia with hyperbaric bupivacaine. *Brit. J. Anaesthesia.* 1982; **54**: 497–500.
53.   Smith T. C. The lumbar spine and subarachnoid block. *Anesthesiol.* 1968; **29**: 60–4.
54.   Wildsmith J. A. W., McClure J. H., Brown D. T., Scott D. B. Effects of posture on the spread of isobaric and hyperbaric amethocaine. *Brit. J. Anaesthesia.* 1981; **53**: 273–8.
55.   McClure J. H., Brown D. T., Wildsmith J. A. W. Effect of injected volume and speed of injection on the spread of spinal anaesthesia with isobaric amethocaine. *Brit. J. Anaesthesia.* 1982; **54**: 917–20.
56.   Logan M. R., McClure J. H., Wildsmith J. A. W. Plain bupivacaine – an unpredictable spinal anaesthetic agent. *Brit. J. Anaesthesia.* 1986; **58**: 292–6.
57.   McCulloch W. J. D., Littlewood D. G. Influence of obesity on spinal

analgesia with isobaric 0.5% bupivacaine. *Brit. J. Anaesthesia.* 1986; **58**: 610–4.

58. Cameron A. E., Arnold R. W., Ghoris M. W., Jamieson V. Spinal analgesia using bupivacaine 0.5% plain. Variations in the extent of block with patient age. *Anaesthesia.* 1981; **36**: 318–22.

59. Pitkanen M., Haapaniemi L., Touminen M., Rosenberg P. H. Influence of age on spinal anaesthesia with isobaric 0.5% bupivacaine. *Brit. J. Anaesthesia.* 1984; **56**: 279–84.

60. Axelsson K. H., Edstrom H. H., Widman G. B. Spinal anaesthesia with glucose free 0.5% bupivacaine – effects of different volumes. *Brit. J. Anaesthesia.* 1984; **56**: 271–8.

61. Chambers W. A., Littlewood D. G., Edstrom H. H., Scott D. B. Spinal anaesthesia with hyperbaric bupivacaine: effects of concentration and volume administered. *Brit. J. Anaesthesia.* 1982; **54**: 75–80.

62. Axelsson K. H., Edstrom H. H., Widman G. B. Spinal anaesthesia with hyperbaric 0.5% bupivacaine – effects of volume. *Acta Anaesth. Scand.* 1982; **26**: 439–45.

6

Clinical use of spinal opioids

M. Morgan

The provision of effective postoperative analgesia is one of the major problems still facing the speciality of anaesthesia today. There are a number of reasons why pain relief after surgery remains less than optimal in many cases. The numbers involved are large and thus any technique used must be relatively simple. Opioids remain the mainstay of treatment, but there is a very large interindividual variation in the response to these drugs. As a result, regimens that fix dosage in advance and which limit the rate of administration for fear of the appearance of side effects are doomed to failure.[1] The regular intramuscular injection given at the discretion of a nurse in a dose chosen by a doctor, without observing its effects, although simple, is largely ineffective. The intravenous route is more efficacious, but side effects are more likely to occur and facilities must be at hand to treat respiratory depression. Patient-controlled analgesia represents a significant advance, but it is not without problems, requiring expensive apparatus that can go wrong, and the limits of dosing are again set by a doctor who will always err on the side of safety.

Regional anaesthetic techniques with local anaesthetics will completely abolish postoperative pain by blockade of the appropriate nerves. Intercostal nerve block can produce several hours analgesia, but repeat injections are hardly feasible and continuous techniques difficult. Varying success has been reported using interpleural local anaesthetics. Epidural analgesia can also completely abolish postoperative pain, but may be associated with a number of potentially serious complications.

Epidural opioids represent an alternative approach to the control of postoperative pain.

Epidural opioids

The discovery of opioid receptors in the spinal cord[2] soon led to the demonstration of the profound analgesic effects of morphine and other opioids when applied directly to the spinal cord of rats. The first report of epidural opioids in man was in 1979 in the treatment of intractable pain[3] and since then they have been used extensively not only in chronic, but also in postoperative and other pain of acute origin.

There are a number of important advantages of using opioids via the epidural route:

1. Analgesia is effective and may be very prolonged, especially with morphine, and can often be achieved with smaller doses than are necessary parenterally. Central depression is therefore less and results in a more cooperative patient who can be mobilized earlier.

2. A large number of drugs of varying duration of action are available for use.

3. There is no autonomic blockade and hence no hypotension, which is a major problem when local anaesthetics are used epidurally.

4. There is no loss of any other modality of sensation and no motor blockade.

5. Accidental intravenous injection results in easily treatable complications and is not likely to have the serious consequences of intravenous local anaesthetics.

6. There is no evidence of tachyphylaxis in the management of postoperative pain with epidural opioids.

7. A specific antagonist is available which will reverse all the associated side effects.

Widespread use of epidural opioids, however, has also revealed a number of disadvantages of the technique that must be taken into account if they are to be used on a large scale in the treatment of postoperative pain. Unlike local anaesthetics, analgesia is not complete, and the large interindividual variation in dose requirements seen with other routes of administration, remains. The incidence of relatively 'minor' side effects is high and they require treatment. Above all, respiratory depression still occurs and although this may appear early due to vascular absorption, it may also be delayed for several hours because of rostral spread within the cerebrospinal fluid (CSF).

Mechanism of action

There is little doubt that the main site of action of epidural opioids is at spinal level. Animal work has shown that intense analgesia was produced in rats by opioids applied locally to the spinal cord and which remained locally. Opioids have been shown *in vitro* to inhibit release of the neurotransmitter associated with nociception[4] and it was suggested that this was via pre-synaptically situated opioid receptors. Opioids have also been shown to antagonize the release of substance P in *in vitro* experiments.[5]

Clinical evidence also supports a spinal site of action, although there is some initial contribution due to systemic absorption. No relationship can be found between quality of analgesia and plasma levels of the various opioids, which are well below the normally accepted analgesic concentrations.[6-9] Volunteer studies in humans have shown that analgesia is present in the lower limbs following lumbar epidural morphine, but not in the upper parts of the body.[10, 11]

Pharmacokinetics

As the main site of action of epidural opioids is on the spinal cord, the drug must initially cross the dura and arachnoid to gain entry to the CSF before passing into the spinal cord. The fate of the drug following epidural injection is going to depend on its physico-chemical properties and in particular its lipid solubility, and is shown diagramatically in Fig. 6.1. The lipid solubilities of some of the commonly used opioid drugs are shown in Table 6.1.

Table 6.1 Octanol: water partition coefficient of different opioids at pH 7.4 (except buprenorphine, which is at pH 6.75).

Drug	Lipid solubility
Morphine	1.42
Pethidine	38.8
Methadone	116
Alfentanil	126
Fentanyl	813
Sufentanil	1778
Buprenorphine	2320

A lipid-soluble drug would rapidly cross the dura into the CSF and would quickly enter the spinal cord. Onset of analgesia would be rapid and of a segmental nature, but of relatively short duration. (An exception would be buprenorphine which, although highly lipid soluble, because of its receptor binding characteristics would be expected to produce prolonged analgesia.) Little drug would remain in the CSF and be available for rostral spread so that the incidence of delayed respiratory depression would be very low. However, as well as crossing the dura rapidly, a fat-soluble drug would also be taken up into the systemic circulation quickly, and dissolve in epidural fat, all of which would be lost for dural transfer.

In contrast, much less of a poorly lipid-soluble drug, e.g. morphine,

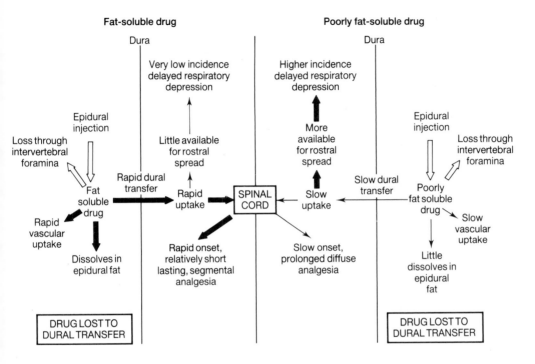

Figure 6.1 Fate of fat-soluble and poorly fat-soluble drug injected into the epidural space. More of the fat-soluble drug is lost to dural transfer. Passage across the dura and entry into the spinal cord is rapid, producing fast onset, segmental analgesia of relatively short duration. Little drug will be available for rostral spread. In contrast, dural transfer of a poorly fat-soluble drug is slow, but more drug will remain available for passage across the dura. Analgesia will be slow in onset, long lasting and of a diffuse nature. More is available for rostral spread and the incidence of complications, particularly delayed respiratory depression, will be higher.

would be lost to dural transfer by vascular uptake and dissolving in epidural fat. Transfer into the CSF and entry into the spinal cord would be slow and the drug would tend to linger in the CSF. Analgesia would be slow in onset and non-segmental. Much more drug would be available for rostral spread and a much higher incidence of delayed respiratory depression compared to more fat soluble drugs can be expected. Duration of analgesia will also be longer with lipophobic drugs.

In *in vitro* experiments involving isolated human dura mater, lipophilicity was not found to be an important factor in determining dural transfer, morphine and the much more fat soluble diamorphine having the same permeabilities.[12] Permeability had a linear relationship to the inverse square root of the molecular weight of the drug, but fentanyl was an exception and crossed the dura faster than expected. It was therefore suggested that molecular shape may be the important factor and that whereas most of the compounds tested had a spherical shape, fentanyl is an extended molecule.

This work suggested that a small molecular weight drug such as morphine would be efficiently transferred across the dura, but this is not borne out clinically. Following epidural injection, peak plasma morphine concentrations occur at about 15 minutes[13,14] and it crosses the dura slowly with peak CSF concentrations occurring between 90 and 120 minutes.[14,15] Disappearance from CSF is prolonged with about 50 per cent still being present at 12 hours. However, the amount of morphine entering CSF after epidural injection is small, the CSF bioavailability being between 2 and 4 per cent.[6, 15] These findings are consistent with the slow onset and long duration of epidural morphine.

Pharmacokinetic and clinical data concerning the fat-soluble diamorphine support the suggestions concerning lipophilic drugs shown in Fig. 6.1. Peak plasma levels of morphine after epidural diamorphine (which is rapidly converted into morphine in the circulation and can't itself be measured in plasma) occur significantly faster and are significantly higher than after epidural mophine.[16] Diamorphine is removed from CSF more rapidly than morphine, with the former having an elimination half-life after 1 mg of 43 minutes compared to 73 minutes after 1 mg of morphine.[17, 18] These studies support the clinical findings of more rapid onset and shorter duration of analgesia of epidural diamorphine compared to morphine, and also lend support to the higher incidence of delayed respiratory depression with the poorly lipid-soluble morphine.

Choice of drug

Epidural opioids produce effective and often prolonged analgesia, although there is little convincing evidence that the quality of analgesia is superior to that produced by the more conventional routes of administration. But the analgesia is achieved with only about 20–40 per cent of the systemic dose of morphine when given epidurally, and only 8 per cent intrathecally.[19] A list of drugs that have been used epidurally in the treatment of postoperative pain, the doses used and the mode of administration are shown in Table 6.2.

Morphine

This is by far the commonest drug used epidurally on a world-wide basis for postoperative pain. It is the least soluble of the opioids and behaves as

Table 6.2 Drugs that have been used epidurally with doses and method of administration

Drug	Method	Dose
Morphine	Bolus	2.0–10.0 mg, 0.1 mg.kg^{-1}
	Infusion	100–400 µg.h^{-1}
Diamorphine	Bolus	0.5–10.0 mg, 0.1 mg.kg^{-1}
Pethidine	Bolus	25.0–100.0 mg, 1.0 mg.kg^{-1}
Methadone	Bolus	4.0–6.0 mg
Hydromorphone	Bolus	1.0 mg
Fentanyl	Bolus	100–200 µg
	Infusion	20–130 µg.h^{-1}
Alfentanil	Bolus	15.0–300 µg.kg^{-1}
	Infusion	200 µg.h^{-1}
Sufentanil	Bolus	15.0–75.0 µg
	Infusion	3.0 µg.kg.$^{-1}$h^{-1}
Lofentanil	Bolus	5.0 µg
Phenoperidine	Bolus	2.0 mg
Buprenorphine	Bolus	60.0–900 µg
Butorphanol	Bolus	1.0–4.0 mg
Nalbuphine	Bolus	10.0 mg
Meptazinol	Bolus	30.0–09.0 mg
Pentazocine	Bolus	0.3 mg.kg^{-1}

(Source: reference 65).

would be expected from Fig. 6.1. Onset of action is slow and it produces prolonged, non-segmental analgesia. The incidence of complications is high due to the persistence of the drug in the CSF and its slow rostral spread. Onset of effective analgesia can often take up to 60 minutes and thus has the disadvantage that more drug might be given in the belief that the original dose was too small and ineffective. The incidence of complications would also increase under these circumstances.[20]

Diamorphine

This is the diacetyl derivative of morphine and considerably less polar. Dural transfer is more rapid with consequent faster appearance of analgesia. Several reports attest to the efficacy of postoperative analgesia following epidural diamorphine, although duration of effect is shorter than morphine; the incidence of complications is lower. The drug enjoys considerable popularity in the UK, but its use is banned in most countries because of its abuse potential.

Pethidine

Pethidine was the first opioid to be used epidurally in the management of postoperative pain.[21] Dural transfer is rapid, and effective analgesia can be expected within 20 minutes of administration. Reported duration of analgesia varies widely, but can be as long as 6–7 hours. Extensive experience with the drug has been reported by Brownridge[22] following gynaecological surgery and Caesarean section, with minimum side effects.

Fentanyl

This is one of the most fat-soluble of the opioid drugs (Table 6.1) and, as would be predicted, produces fast onset, short duration analgesia following a single bolus injection. Its properties make it an ideal drug for use of infusion and there are numerous reports concerning its efficacy when used in this manner. Its relatively short duration of action means that side effects appear more rapidly and that the risks of delayed effects are minimal. Late respiratory depression is therefore unlikely to be a problem and discharge from an area of high surveillance can be safely achieved more quickly than after a drug such as morphine.

Buprenorphine

Buprenorphine is an extremely fat-soluble drug and entry into the CSF and spinal cord is rapid. However, because of its slow receptor kinetics and high receptor affinity, onset of analgesia is relatively slow and akin to morphine, and duration of analgesia is much longer than the other fat-soluble agents, being in the region of 8–10 hours.[23] Very prolonged analgesia, as is sometimes noted after morphine, has been reported.

Virtually all the currently available opioids have been used epidurally (Table 6.2) but there have been few comparative studies. No differences would be expected in the quality of analgesia, but variations will be seen in the speed of onset, duration of analgesia and incidence of complications. Thus, in doses which are generally regarded as being equipotent parenterally, no difference was found in the quality of analgesia but only in duration, following epidural administration of morphine 6 mg (12.3 hours), methadone 6 mg (8.7 hours), pethidine 60 mg (6.6 hours) and fentanyl 60μg (5.1 hours).[24] No difference in the quality of analgesia exists between epidural morphine and diamorphine.[16]

The choice of drug will therefore rest with individual preference and availability, taking into account the nature and source of the pain, the pharmacokinetic and pharmacodynamic properties, the incidence of complications, the facilities for patient management postoperatively and the method of administration, by bolus injection or continuous infusion.

Dose of drug

It was well known that there is a large interindividual variation in the response to opioid drugs and that this is the reason for failure of regimens giving fixed doses parenterally on an on-demand basis for the management of postoperative pain. Such interpatient variation also applies when the epidural route is used and care must be taken not to fall into the trap of assuming that one dose will suit everyone. Analgesia can usually be attained by lower doses than conventional intramuscular amounts, but failure rates of 10–20 per cent when treating postoperative pain with epidural opioids[25] are probably the result of inadequate dosage.

Despite the fact that the technique has been used for ten years, there have been few dose-finding studies. The epidural dose necessary to produce effective analgesia postoperatively will vary according to the nature and site of surgery. Morphine 2 mg has been reported as producing excellent analgesia after lower limb orthopaedic surgery, with no benefit being obtained from increasing the dose up to 8 mg.[26] Similar results were found by other workers, who also found the incidence of complications increased with increasing dose.[27] After abdominal and thoracic surgery, morphine 2 mg was found to be ineffective[28,29] and 6 mg was required to produce adequate analgesia.[30] Long-lasting pain relief after similar surgery was produced by buprenorphine 300 µg and 900 µg, there being no additional benefit from the larger dose.[23]

It is obvious from the literature that the majority of workers use a fixed dose of opioids epidurally when treating postoperative pain, and this is no doubt the reason for the 10–20 per cent failure rate already mentioned. In order to achieve optimal analgesia the dose of drug must be titrated against the individual patient's needs. Bromage, Camporesi and Chestnut[31] found that the dose of epidural morphine necessary to produce adequate pain relief after upper abdominal surgery was very similar to the intravenous dose. Analgesia lasted much longer with the former route and there was significantly less central depression. With drugs of slow onset, care must be taken to allow adequate time for assessing efficacy before additional doses are given in order to avoid overdose and consequent high incidence of side-effects. The latency time for morphine can be as long as an hour, particularly when given into the lumbar epidural space to relieve pain from upper abdominal and thoracic incisions. When using infusions, again the rate must be adjusted to the patient's needs; an infusion rate of fentanyl between 80 and 130 µg.h^{-1} was necessary to provide adequate analgesia following abdominal aortic surgery.[32]

A comparison of patient controlled analgesia via the epidural route after abdominal surgery revealed no difference in the quality of pain relief between morphine and pethidine.[7] Morphine consumption averaged 0.52 mg.h^{-1} compared to pethidine 18.0 mg.h^{-1}, an equi-analgesic dose relationship of 1:35, which is quite different from the parenteral 1:10 relationship. The interindividual drug consumption in this study was considerable, such that the authors could not recommend a standard dose of epidural morphine or pethidine for analgesia of a predictable duration and with a minimum of adverse effects.

Site of injection

As illustrated in Fig. 6.1, a poorly lipid-soluble drug like morphine would be expected to produce diffuse analgesia and therefore the site of injection into the epidural space is unlikely to be critical in terms of optimum analgesia. There are now several reports in the literature attesting to the efficacy of lumbar epidural morphine following upper abdominal and thoracic surgery.[6, 33, 34] A long latency can be expected when morphine is used in this way, and a larger diluent volume, e.g. 10–15 ml, should be used. Even caudal morphine can produce effective analgesia after paediatric cardiac surgery.[35]

Again from Fig. 6.1, the rapid penetration of the neuraxis by the fat-soluble agents would be expected to result in a more discrete segmental analgesia. There are numerous reports of thoracic epidural fentanyl producing excellent analgesia following thoracic and upper abdominal surgery. Placement of thoracic epidural catheters is more difficult than lumbar and potentially more dangerous in terms of damage to the spinal cord. Although studied in much fewer cases, lumbar epidural fentanyl has been used effectively to relieve pain after thoracotomy.[36] A greater initial diluent volume is used by the lumbar route, 1–2 µg.kg^{-1} being given in 18 ml instead of 10 ml when given into the thoracic epidural space. To date, no prospective controlled studies have been performed to confirm or refute the hypothesis that the fat-soluble opioids produce segmental analgesia and require to be given into the appropriate area. Similarly, studies comparing lumbar and thoracic fentanyl for upper abdominal and thoracic incisions have not yet been done.

Existing evidence suggests that better analgesia is obtained if the opioid is given epidurally before the onset of pain.[27, 37] Morphine [38, 39] and diamorphine[40] given epidurally prior to surgery reduce opioid require-ments in the immediate postoperative period. An epidural catheter should therefore be placed before surgery or at the end of the procedure and the opioid given prior to the patient awakening. Controversy exists as to whether the catheter should be sited once the patient is anaesthetized[41] or whilst awake, when potential trauma to the spinal cord would be obvious immediately.[42] It is up to the individual anaesthetist to decide which they think best.

Complications of epidural opioids

The nature and incidence of the complications following epidural opioids will have an important bearing on the choice of drug to be used and on the management of patients in the postoperative period. Minor side-effects are common and can be very distressing for the patient, while the more serious life-threatening complication, respiratory depression to the point of apnoea, is much rarer.

Nausea and vomiting

This side-effect cannot be divorced from the use of opioid drugs and an incidence of around 30 per cent can be expected. This is particularly distressing in the presence of a thoracic or abdominal incision and some form of treatment will be necessary. The incidence can be reduced with naloxone, but prophylactic use of the latter does not abolish the appearance of side-effects and may affect the quality of analgesia.[33] Transdermal hyoscine is effective in reducing nausea and vomiting after epidural morphine.[43]

Pruritus

This is another common and extremely distressing side-effect and the reported incidence varies widely in different series. Opinions differ as to whether it is dose related following morphine; it can also occur with all the other drugs. The itching is not confined to the segmental area of action of the drug, but also occurs around the head and neck. The mechanism is unknown, but there is no evidence that it is due to histamine release since it also occurs with fentanyl which does not have the latter property.

Urinary retention

Epidural morphine, irrespective of dose, results in a marked relaxation of the detrusor muscle shortly after injection, with an increase in bladder capacity and consequent urinary retention.[44] The effect lasts up to 16 hours. As little change is seen after intravenous or intramuscular morphine, a spinal action of epidural morphine is favoured. The effects are promptly reversed with naloxone. Urinary retention can occur in up to 90 per cent of men given epidural morphine and it is of considerable importance in those who do not have an indwelling urinary catheter. It is probably the most troublesome complication occurring after spinal opioids.

Neurological damage

This is always a concern following epidural and intrathecal analgesia, but there is no evidence that opioids used by these routes cause damage to nerve tissue. Drug preparations containing preservatives, however, should not be used as these may be neurotoxic, for example chlorocresol, phenol and formaldehyde.

Respiratory depression

The initial hope that respiratory depression would not be a feature of epidurally applied opioids has been unfounded. It can occur soon after drug administration due to systemic absorption, or it can be delayed for several hours due to rostral spread of drug in the CSF. The former is usually associated with the more fat-soluble drugs, while delayed depression usually, but not invariably, follows use of lipophobic agents, particularly morphine. A list of drugs associated with respiratory depression and the time of occurrence after epidural administration is shown in Table 6.3.

Table 6.3 Drugs which have been followed by clinically evident respiratory depression after epidural use, with time of appearance.

Drug	Dose	Time
Morphine	2.0–10.0 mg	30 min–16.5 hours
Diamorphine	2.0–10.0 mg	20 min– 4.5 hours
Pethidine	50.0–100.0 mg	5–30 min
Methadone	4.0–6.0 mg	20 min–4.0 hours
Hydromorphone	1.0 mg	4.5 hours
Sufentanil	50.0 μg	5–15 min
Fentanyl	100.0 μg	30–100 min[66]–4 hours

(Source: reference 65)

Experimental work in primates found that morphine was maximally concentrated in the medulla 6 hours after intrathecal injection.[45] In a series of experiments on sheep, morphine, methadone and sucrose were injected simultaneously into the lumbar epidural space. Morphine and sucrose levels peaked maximally in cisternal CSF at about 3 hours, but no methadone was detectable up to 5 hours.[46] Because of obvious difficulties, information on spread of opioids in the CSF in humans is markedly limited. Cousins and his colleagues[21] showed rapid transfer of pethidine into the CSF after epidural administration in postoperative patients. Morphine concentrations in cervical CSF peaked 2–3 hours after injection into the lumbar epidural space, while pethidine peaked earlier and at a higher concentration than morphine. Two hours after injection, pethidine concentrations were lower than morphine.[47]

Volunteer work in humans confirms that maximum respiratory depression after epidural morphine occurs between 6 and 10 hours, while evidence of depression can persist for up to 24 hours.[48, 49] There is also evidence that the respiratory depression is of a biphasic nature, occurring at 1–2 hours because of systemic absorption and again at around 8 hours due to rostral spread in the CSF.[50]

The lipophilic drugs diffuse rapidly into the circulation and across the dura, and the CSF levels fall rapidly, limiting cephalad spread (Fig. 6.1). Confirmatory evidence exists in man. Diamorphine concentrations fall more rapidly in CSF than morphine,[17, 18] while pethidine disappears from CSF about four times faster than morphine.[15] It is probable that the other fat-soluble opioids behave in a similar way, although there is no direct evidence in man. Following these drugs, respiratory depression usually occurs within 30 minutes of administration. However, delayed respiratory depression has been reported after diamorphine, methadone, hydromorphine and fentanyl. It should be pointed out that the report of the latter hardly accords with most anaesthetists definition of clinically relevant respiratory depression.[51]

Experimental work has shown that fentanyl 200 μg given epidurally to volunteers results in a significant decrease in the CO_2 response curve for up to 2 hours.[52] Until recently, significant respiratory depression has not been reported after fentanyl, although the author has seen patients with respiratory rates of 6 breaths minute^{-1} whilst receiving epidural fentanyl at a rate of 1μg.kg^{-1} h^{-1} for postoperative analgesia. However, an authenticated case of complete apnoea has now been described 100 minutes after fentanyl 100 μg has been injected epidurally in a young, previously healthy woman. This patient would have been regarded as being of extremely low risk of developing this complication. Reports of the problem after pethidine are rare, but severe early depression, including respiratory arrest has been seen after sufentanil[53] and alfentanil.[54] Buprenorphine, which is one of the most soluble of the opioids (Table 6.1), has been associated with early and persistent respiratory depression in postoperative patients,[23] and in volunteers has been shown to cause a biphasic depression in the respiratory response to CO_2, indicating that rostral spread in the CSF does occur.[55] Butorphanol also causes a prolonged depressant effect as judged by CO_2 response curves.[56] The whole field of respiratory depression following spinal opioids has been extensively reviewed recently.[57]

In most cases, respiratory depression usually develops gradually over a period of 15–20 minutes and is accompanied by gradual loss of consciousness. Respiratory inductance plethysmography has shown that there is a high incidence of abnormal respiratory patterns following use of epidural morphine for postoperative pain relief.[20] These alterations were subtle and insidious in onset and of unpredictable duration.

The true incidence of clinically significant respiratory depression after epidural morphine is not known, and has varied between 0.09 per cent and 3.1 per cent in reported large series. Large prospective trials are necessary to determine the frequency of this potentially lethal complication. However, there are a number of factors that seem to determine the appearance of delayed respiratory depression (Table 6.4).[58] Particularly important is the concomitant use of parenteral opioids or other central depressant drugs to patients who have not been chronically exposed to narcotics. A number of factors that encourage rostral spread of drugs in the CSF, such as coughing, vomiting, straining, artificial ventilation, are impossible to control in the postoperative patient. This could account for the different incidences of respiratory depression and the timing of its appearance in different series.

Table 6.4 Factors predisposing to the developing of respiratory depression after extradural opioids.[58]

Advanced age
Use of water soluble drugs such as morphine
Concomitant use of parenteral opioids or other centrally acting depressant
   drugs
Lack of tolerance to opioids
Increased intrathoracic pressure e.g. artificial ventilation, coughing,
   vomiting
Large doses
Use of thoracic route

Epidural opioids have now been in use for over ten years, and although properly controlled prospective studies with large numbers are required to elucidate the true incidence of respiratory depression after the various drugs, some conclusions can now be drawn which will influence the management of patients when the technique is used:

1.   The appearance of respiratory depression is unpredictable.

2.   The incidence after morphine, and particularly the occurrence of delayed respiratory depression, make it an unsuitable drug for epidural use for postoperative pain.

3.   Respiratory depression is most likely to occur within 1 hour of administration of the fat-soluble drugs. Although rare, delayed respiratory depression can occur and must be taken into account when these drugs are used.

4.   All opioid drugs have the propensity to cause respiratory depression when used epidurally.

Management of epidural opioids postoperatively

That epidural opioids produce effective analgesia in doses smaller than those given parenterally, with the attendant benefits of less central depression, greater cooperation and mobility, is not questionable. For optimum analgesia the first dose should be given before the patient has regained consciousness. Thereafter it is imperative that the dose be titrated against the patients' needs. Care must be taken with drugs of slow onset lest an overdose be given in the erroneous belief that the first dose was ineffective. The shorter acting agents, like fentanyl and alfentanil, are best given by continuous infusion, but again must be adjusted to each patient's requirements. Experience with patient-controlled analgesia via the epidural route is as yet limited, but warrants full investigation.

The price paid for this excellent analgesia, however, is a high incidence of side-effects. Nausea, vomiting and pruritus are common, and instructions must be given to the nursing staff with regard to treatment. Urinary retention is problematical in non-catheterized patients and will require immediate treatment.

The major concern relating to the use of epidural opioids is respiratory depression, and particularly the possibility of its delayed appearance. The question that requires to be answered is whether it is safe to manage these patients on an ordinary ward postoperatively or whether they require to be nursed in an area where more intensive surveillance is available. The incidence of delayed respiratory depression after morphine is such that most agree that close observation is required for up to 24 hours after its use. Nevertheless a survey in Sweden revealed that 18 per cent of anaesthetic departments returned patients to an ordinary ward with no special observations after epidural morphine.[59]

The situation is much less clear when it comes to use of fat-soluble drugs. Brownridge[22] has used pethidine 50 mg in some 2000 women following Caesarean section and gynaecological surgery, with minimum complications, the patients being returned to an ordinary ward. The author has been told by colleagues that they routinely use diamorphine or fentanyl after Caesarean section under epidural anaesthesia and return the patients to an ordinary ward, and the practice would appear to be widespread. The literature indicates that morphine is also frequently used in these patients.

Those who have undergone Caesarean section or gynaecological surgery form a low risk group with regard to the development of respiratory depression. They are generally young, have undergone a lower abdominal operations and have no chest disease. But even so, is it justifiable to take no special precautions in these patients? Depressed responsiveness to CO_2 has been demonstrated for up to 24 hours after 5 mg epidural morphine to post-Caesarean-section mothers.[56] Kotelko and colleagues[60] gave naloxone to one of 276 mothers after Caesarean section who had received 5 mg epidural morphine, while others have reported incidences after this operation of 4 per 1000[61] and 2 per 3000.[62] It has been pointed out that if a successful series of 1000 cases has been achieved, the 99.9 per cent probability that the next patient would be all right would be 145:1.[42] Is this an acceptable risk in the treatment of postoperative pain?

Monitoring

The evidence that exists at the moment indicates that patients in receipt of epidural opioids require more intensive observation than can be provided on an ordinary general ward.

Observations of respiratory rate on an hourly basis is totally inadequate. Monitoring should be continuous with particular attention being paid to any trends that occur, as the aim is to prevent the development of respiratory depression rather than to treat it once it has occurred. Such monitoring should be simple, not require patient cooperation, be non-invasive and applicable to several patients simultaneously. This could best be provided by constant supervision by the nursing staff. Respiratory inductance plethysmography is not practical as a routine, while apnoea alarms merely inform that an event that should have been prevented has happened. End-tidal CO_2 monitors are valuable but are not available in sufficiently large numbers in the UK to be used for postoperative monitoring. Transcutaneous CO_2 electrodes still await critical analysis in a large series to establish their reliability.

Most would advocate the use of pulse oximetry in these patients, but their accuracy can be affected by many factors. Furthermore, arterial hypoxaemia is a feature of the postoperative period and and an oxygen mask accidentally slipping off the face will result in desaturation and cause the instrument to alarm. Frequent occurrence of such an event will eventually result in the alarm being ignored. As well as respiration, conscious level must also be monitored in these patients, and again it is the trend that is important.

The necessary monitoring thus requires the immediate availability of trained personnel in an area of high dependency or intensive care. Such personnel must be allowed to give intravenous injections, as the respiratory depression produced by epidural opioids is immediately reversed by intravenous naloxone. The latter must therefore be instantly available wherever these patients are nursed.

Two groups have described the provision of an acute pain service for the management of postoperative pain by anaesthetists.[63, 64] Both provide 24 hour cover and stress the importance of education of nursing and non-anaesthetic medical staff in the care of patients receiving epidural opioids. As the incidence of minor complications is high, instructions are given to the nursing staff as to their treatment. Because of the danger of respiratory depression, medication is only prescribed by anaesthetists. The services are expensive in terms of manpower.

Busch and Steadman[64] have used this approach for a number of years in treating postoperative pain on general medical and surgical wards with epidural morphine, with no serious sequelae. Ready and his colleagues[63] also use epidural morphine on ordinary wards and laid down the criteria for when a respiratory monitor was to be used. These are:

1. Patients older than 50 years.
2. ASA status other than I or II.
3. Thoracic or upper abdominal surgery.
4. Surgery greater than 4 hours duration.
5. When narcotics or other long-acting central depressants had been used during surgery.
6. When the dose of morphine was greater than 6. mg epidurally or 0.5 mg intrathecally.

Monitors were not required in areas of continuous nursing surveillance. These criteria were only guidelines and monitors could be used at any time on the discretion of the medical or nursing staff.

At the time of their report, epidural morphine had been used in 623 patients, and delayed respiratory depression occurred in four. All these satisfied the criteria for close respiratory monitoring. It is noteworthy that the arterial carbon dioxide tension in these patients ranged from 8.4–12.7 kPa (63–95 mmHg) and was measured because of alterations in conscious level. All these patients were in the 'high risk' group with regard to the development of respiratory depression and presumably respiratory monitors were used, but the complication was not prevented.

Intrathecal opioids

The main factor determining analgesia by spinal opioids is the concentration of the drug in the CSF. It would thus seem much more logical to inject the drug directly intrathecally and avoid the problems of systemic absorption of epidurally administered drug. Prolonged and effective postoperative analgesia can be achieved with much less drug than by other routes.[19]

Problems of maintaining a catheter intrathecally for up to several days means that this route is not satisfactory for providing prolonged analgesia after surgery. The incidence of complications is also higher than after epidural injection, particularly respiratory depression.[65] The problem of post-lumbar-puncture headache must also be considered. Although the method is used for patients who are admitted to an intensive care unit and require artificial ventilation postoperatively, e.g. following cardiac surgery, it has found much less favour in the UK than epidural opioids.

Conclusions

Epidural opioids can provide excellent and prolonged analgesia post-operatively in doses which are often much lower than by conventional routes. Nevertheless their use is accompanied by a relatively high incidence of 'minor' side effects which require treatment. The major problem of their use remains that of respiratory depression and its unpredictability. High-risk patients are usually easily identifiable, but there is the occasional patient, with no apparent risk factors, who develops respiratory depression. Adequate monitoring of these patients is therefore essential in the postoperative period; this is time consuming and heavily demanding on nursing and medical staff. Until the results of large prospective studies on the use of the various opioids epidurally for postoperative analgesia are known, it is difficult to justify the management of these patients on an ordinary ward after surgery.

References

1. Bullingham R. E. S. Optimum management of postoperative pain. *Drugs* 1985; **29**: 376–86.
2. LaMotte C., Pert C. B., Snyder S. H. Opiate receptor binding in primate spinal cord: distribution and changes after dorsal root section.*Brain Res.* 1976; **112**: 407–12.
3. Behar M., Magora F., Olshwang D., Davidson J. T. Epidural morphine in treatment of pain. *Lancet* 1979; **1**: 527–8.
4. Jessell T. M., Iverson L. L. Opiate analgesics inhibit substance P release from rat trigeminal nucleus. *Nature (London)* 1977; **268**: 549–51.
5. Yaksh T. L., Jessell T. M., Gause R., Mudge A. W., Leeman S. E. Intrathecal morphine inhibits substance P release from mammalian spinal cord *in vivo*. *Nature (London)* 1980; **286**: 155–7.
6. Nordberg G., Hedner T., Mellstrand T., Borg L. Pharmacokinetics of epidural morphine in man. *Eur. J. Clin. Pharmacol.* 1984; **26**: 233–7
7. Sjostrom S., Hartvig D., Tamsen A. Patient controlled analgesia with epidural morphine or pethidine. *Brit. J. Anaesthesia* 1988; 60 358–66.
8. Weddel S. J., Ritter R. R. Serum levels following epidural administration of morphine and correlation with relief of postsurgical pain. *Anesthesiol* 1981; **54**: 210–4.
9. Youngstrom P. C., Cowan R. I., Sutheimer C., Eastwood D. W., Yu J. C. M. Pain relief and plasma concentrations from epidural and intramuscular morphine in post-Cesarean patients. *Anesthesiol.* 1982; **57**: 404–9.

10. Torda T. A., Pybus D. A., Lisberman H., Clark M., Crawford M. Experimental comparison of extradural and i.m. morphine. *Brit. J. Anaesthesia* 1980; **52**: 939–43.
11. Thomson W. R., Smith P. R., Hirst M., Varkey G. P., Knill R. L. Regional analgesic effect of epidural morphine in volunteers. *Can. Anaesth. Soc. J.* 1981; **28**: 530–6.
12. Moore R. A., Bullingham R. E. S., McQuay H. J., Hand C. W., Aspel C. B., Allen M. G., Thomas D. Dural permeability to narcotics: *in vitro* determination and application to extradural administration. *Brit. J. Anaesthesia.* 1982; 1117–28.
13. Nordberg G. Pharmacokinetic aspects of spinal morphine analgesia. *Acta Anaestheiol. Scand.* 1984; **28**: (Suppl. 79): 6–38.
14. Nordberg G., Hedner T., Mellstrand T., Dahlstrom B. Pharmacokinetic aspect of epidural morphine analgesia. *Anesthesiol.* 1983; **58**: 545–51.
15. Sjostrom S., Hartvig P., Persson M. P., Tamsen A. Pharmocokinetics of epidural morphine and meperidine in humans. *Anesthesiol.* 1987; **67**: 877–88.
16. Watson J., Moore A., McQuay H., Teddy P., Balwin D., Allen M., Bullingham R. E. S. Plasma morphine concentrations and analgesic effects of lumbar extradural morphine and heroin. *Anesthesia and Analgesia* 1984; **63**: 129–34.
17. Moore R. A., Bullingham R. E. S., McQuay H., Allen M., Baldwin D., Cole A. Spinal fluid kinetics of morphine and heroin. *Clin. Pharmacol. and Ther.* 1984; **35**: 40–5.
18. Kotob H. I. M., Hand C. W., Moore R. A., Evans P. J. D., Wells J., Rubin A. P., McQuay H. J. Intrathecal morphine and heroin in humans: six hour drug levels in spinal fluid and plasma. *Anesthesia and Analgesia* 1986; **65**: 718–22.
19. Dahlstrom B. Pharmacokinetics and pharmacodynamics of epidural and intrathecal morphine. *Int. Anesthesiol. Clin.* 1986; **25**: 29–42.
20. Sandler A. N., Chovaz P., Whiting W., Respiratory depression following epidural morphine: a clinical study. *Can. Anaesth. Soc. J.* 1986; **33**: 542–9.
21. Cousins M. J., Mather L. E., Glinn C. J., Wilson P. R., Graham J. R. Selective spinal analgesia. *Lancet* 1979; **1**: 1141–2.
22. Brownridge P. Epidural and intrathecal opiates for postoperative pain relief. *Anaesthesia* 1983; **38**: 74–5.
23. Gundersen R. Y., Anderson R., Narverus G. Postoperative pain relief with high-dose epidural buprenorphine: a double-blind study. *Acta Anaesthesiol. Scand.* 1986; **30**: 664–7.
24. Torda T. A., Pybus D. A. Comparison of four narcotic analgesics for extradural analgesia. *Brit. J. Anaesthesia* 1982; **54**: 291–5.
25. Bilsback P., Rolly G., Tampubolon O. Efficacy of the extradural administration of lofentanil, buprenorphine or saline in the management of postoperative pain. *Brit. J. Anaesthesia* 1985; **57**: 943–8.
26. Martin S., Salbaing J., Blaise G., Tetrault J-P., Tetrault L. Epidural morphine for postoperative pain relief: a dose-response curve. *Anesthesiol.* 1982; **56**: 423–6.
27. Lanz E., Kehrberger E., Theiss D. Epidural morphine: a clinical double-blind study of dose. *Anesthesia and Analgesia* 1985; **64**: 786–91.
28. Crawford R., Batra M. S., Fox F. Epidural morphine dose response for postoperative analgesia. *Anesthsiol.* 1981; **55**: A150.

29.   Rutter D. V., Skewes D. G., Morgan M. Extradural opioids for post-operative analgesia. A double-blind comparison of pethidine, fentanyl and morphine. *Brit. J. Anaesthesia* 1981; **53**: 914–20.

30.   Stenseth R., Sellevold O., Brievik H. Extradural morphine for post-operative pain: experience with 1085 patients. *Acta Anaesthesiol. Scand.* 1985; **29**: 148–56.

31.   Bromage P. R., Camporesi E., Chestnut D. Epidural narcotics for post-operative analgesia. *Anesthesia and Analgesia* 1980; **59**: 473–80.

32.   Bell S. D., Levette A., Larijani G. E. The use of continuous lumbar epidural fentanyl or postoperative pain relief in abdominal aortic aneurysms. *Anesthesiol.* 1987; **67**: A234.

33.   Gowan J. D., Hurtig J. B., Fraser R. A., Torbicki E., Kitts J. Naloxone infusion after prophylactic epidural morphine: effects on incidence of postoperative side-effects and quality of analgesia. *Can. J. Anaesthesia* 1988; **35**: 143–8.

34.   Nordberg G., Mellstrand T., Borg L., Hedner T. Extradural morphine: influence of adrenaline admixture. *Brit. J. Anaesthesia.* 1986; **58**: 589–604.

35.   Rosen K., Rosen D., Bank E. Caudal morphine for post-op pain control in children undergoing cardiac surgery. *Anesthesiol.* 1987; **67**: A510.

36.   Benumoff J. L. Management of postoperative pain. In: Benumoff J. L., *Anaesthesia for Thoracic Surgery.* Philadelphia, WB Sunders 1987; 467–76.

37.   Chambers W. A., Sinclair C. J., Scott D. B. Extradural morphine for pain after surgery. *Brit. J. Anaesthesia* 1981; **52**: 921–5.

38.   Gurel A., Unal N., Elevi M., Eren A. Epidural morphine for post-operative pain relief in anorectal surgery. *Anesthesia and Analgesia* 1986; **65**: 499–502.

39.   Rutberg H., Hakanson E., Anderberg B., Jorfeldt L., Martensson J., Schildt B. Effects of extradural administration of morphine or bupivacaine on the endocrine response to upper abdominal surgery. *Brit. J. Anaesthesia* 1984; **56**: 233–38.

40.   Normandale J. P., Schmulian C., Paterson J. L., Burrin J., Morgan M., Hall G. M. Epidural diamorphine and the metabolic response to upper abdominal surgery. *Brit. J. Anaesthesia* 985; **40**: 748–53.

41.   Gough J. D., Williams A. B., Vaughan R. S., Khalil J. F., Butchart E. G. The control of post-thoracotomy pain. A comparative evaluation of thoracic epidural fentanyl infusions and cryo-analgesia. *Anaesthesia* 1988; **43**: 780–3.

42.   Bromage P. R. The control of post-thoracotomy pain. *Anaesthesia* 1989: **44**: 445.

43.   Loper K. A., Ready B. L., Dorman B. H. Prophylactic transdermal scopolamine patches reduce nausea in postoperative patients receiving epidural morphine. *Anesthesia and Analgesia* 1989; **68**: 144–6.

44.   Rawal N., Mollefors K., Axelsson K., Lingardh G., Widman P. An experimental study of urodynamic effects of epidural morphine and naloxone reversal. *Anesthesia and Analgesia* 1983; **62**: 641–7.

45.   Gregory M. A., Brock-Utne J. G., Bux S., Downing J. W. Morphine concentration in brain and spinal cord after subarachnoid morphine injection in baboons. *Anesthesia and Analgesia* 1985; **64**: 929–32.

46.   Payne R., Inturrisi C. E. CSF distribution of morphine, methadone and sucrose after intrathecal injection. *Life SC.* 1985; **37**: 1137–44.

47.   Gourlay G. K., Cherry D. A., Plummer J. L., Armstrong P. J., Cousins

M. J. The influence of drug polarity on the absorption of opioid drugs into CSF and subsequent cephalad migration following epidural administration: application to morphine and pethidine. *Pain 1987;* **31**: 297–305.

48. Camporesi E. N., Nielsen C. H., Bromage P. R., Durant P. A. C. Ventilatory CO_2 sensitivity after intravenous and epidural morphine in volunteers. *Anesthesia and Analgesia* 1983; **62**: 633–40.

49. Knill R. L., Clement J. L., Thomson W. R. Epidural morphine causes delayed and prolonged ventilatory depression. *Can. Anaesth. Soc. J.* 1981; **28**: 537–43.

50. Kafer E. R., Brown J. T., Scott D., Findlay J. W. A., Butz R. F., Teeple E., Ghia J. B. Biphasic depression of ventilatory responses to CO_2 following epidural morphine. *Anesthesiol* 1983; **58**: 418–27.

51. Parker E. O., Brookshire G. L., Bartel S. J., Menard R. G., Culverhous E. D., Ault L. C. Effects of epinephine on epidural fentanyl, sufentanil and hydromorphone for postoperative analgesia. *Anesthesiol* 1985; **63**: A235.

52. Negre I., Gueneron J. P., Ecoffey C., Penon C., Gross J. B., Levron J-C., Samii K. Ventilatory response to carbon dioxide after intramuscular and epidural fentanyl. *Anesthesia and Analgesia* 1987; **66**: 707–10.

53. Whiting W. G., Sandler A. N., Lau L. C., Chovaz P. M. Analgesic and respiratory effects of epidural sufentanil in post-thoracotomy patients. *Anesthesiol.* 1988; **69**: 36–42.

54. Chauvin M., Salbaing J., Perrin D., Levron J. C., Viars P. Clinical assessment and plasma pharmacokinetics associated with intramuscular or extradural alfentanil. *Brit. J. Anaesthesia* 1985; **57**: 886–91.

55. Molke-Jensen F., Jensen F-H., Holk I. K., Ravnborg M. Prolonged and biphasic respiratory depression following epidural buprenorphine. *Anaesthesia* 1987; **42**: 470–5.

56. Abboud T. K., Moore M., Zhu J., Murakawa K., Minehart M., Longhitano M., Terrasi J., Klepper I. D., Choi Y., Kimball S., Chu G. Epidural butorphanol or morphine for the relief of post Cesarean section pain: ventilatory responses to carbon dioxide. *Anesthesia and Analgesia* 1987; **66**: 887–93.

57. Etches R. C., Sandler A. N., Daley M. D. Respiratory depression and spinal opioids. *Can. J. of Anaesth.* 1989; **36**: 165–185.

58. Cousins M. J., Mather L. E. Intrathecal and epidural administration of opioids. *Anesthesiol* 1984; **61**: 276–310.

59. Rawal N., Arner S., Gustaffson L. L., Alvi R. Present state of extradural and intrathecal opioid analgesia in Sweden. A nationwide follow up study. *Brit. J. Anaesthesia* 1987; **59**: 791–799.

60. Kotelko D. M., Dailey P., Shnider S. M., Rosen M. A., Hughes S. C., Brixgys R. V. Epidural morphine for analgesia after Cesarean delivery. *Obst. and Gynecol.* 1984; **63**: 409–13.

61. Leicht C. H., Hugher S. C., Dailey P. A., Shnider S. M., Rosen M. A. Epidural morphine sulfate after Cesarean section : a prospective report of 1000 patients. *Anesthesiol.* 1986; **65**: A366.

62. McMorland G. H., Douglas J. D. Epidural morphine for postoperative analgesia. *Can. Anaesth. Soc. J.* 1986; **33**: 115–6.

63. Ready L. B., Oden R., Chadwick H. S., Benedetti C., Rook G. A., Caplan R., Wild L. M. Development of an anaesthesiology-based postoperative pain management service. *Anesthesiol.* 1988; **68**: 100–6.

64.   Busch E. H., Stedman P. M. Epidural morphine for postoperative pain on medical-surgical wards – a clinical review. *Anaesthesiol.* 1987; **67**: 101–4.

65.   Morgan M. The rational use of intrathecal and extradural opioids. *Brit. J. Anaesthesia* , In press.

66.   Brockway M. S., Noble D. W., Sharwood-Smith G. H., McClure J. H. Profound respiratory depression after extradural fentanyl. *Brit. J. Anaesthesia* 1990; **64**: 243–45.

7

Management of continuous epidural block

A. Lee

Continuous infusion of a local anaesthetic into the epidural space for postoperative analgesia was described over thirty years ago.[1] Until recently it was a technique employed by a few enthusiasts in specialized centres, but now an increasing number of anaesthetists use such infusions for pain relief in labour or after surgery. The inadequacies of conventional analgesic regimes, the availability of reliable infusion devices and increased experience with epidural techniques have all contributed to more widespread use.

An epidural block may be maintained by one of several methods and the term continuous epidural analgesia may refer to a block that is continued intermittently rather than being truly continuous. Repeated bolus administration of local anaesthetic and/or opioid drugs may be used and self-administration with a patient-controlled analgesia device has been described.[2, 3] In this chapter the term continuous epidural analgesia will imply a fixed rate infusion using a volumetric pump or syringe driver.

The main attributes of continuous epidural analgesia are:

1. Prevention rather than intermittent relief of pain.
2. Better haemodynamic stability than with intermittent epidural injections of local anaesthetic.
3. Reduction of staff time spent checking and administering intermittent injections. This allows more time for direct patient care. The need for nursing *observation* of the patient is in no way reduced.

Before discussing the management of continuous epidural blockade, the drugs and the potential problems associated with their use should be considered. The type of surgery, the equipment available and the degree of postoperative supervision may influence the choice of method. Experience with different techniques enables the anaesthetist to tailor the analgesic regimen to the patient, so achieving the maximum efficacy with the minimum risk.

Agents

Many drugs have been tried epidurally in man for postoperative analgesia.[4, 5] At present, practical and effective continuous epidural analgesia implies the use of a local anaesthetic, an opioid or a combination of the two.

Bupivacaine is the local anaesthetic of choice because systemic accumulation of drug is slow with the doses required to maintain an adequate block, and an infusion may be used safely for several days with little risk of systemic toxicity.[6, 7]

There is a wide range of opioid drugs available for continuous epidural administration. Morphine remains the most commonly used drug despite its slow onset, long duration of action and known potential for late respiratory depression.[8] Fentanyl, diamorphine and other lipophilic drugs such as alfentanil or sufentanil may be more suitable, although these drugs are not without potential problems. Pethidine has some local anaesthetic action and might be expected to produce better analgesia than other opioids, but clinical studies do not support this.[9] The place of agonist-antagonist drugs for postoperative epidural analgesia is not yet well defined.[10, 11]

Combined local anaesthetic and opioid infusions should have a major role in the provision of analgesia after abdominal surgery. There are significant advantages to be gained from the use of a mixture, notably profound analgesia and increased safety.[12, 13] This latter aspect will be discussed more fully later.

Potential problems

Complications may occur with a properly functioning epidural infusion or when the solution is infused incorrectly into another anatomical site. Side effects with a correctly sited catheter may occur as a result of the patient's condition, the type of surgery or complications from surgery e.g. postoperative haemorrhage, equipment faults, or human error in setting up the equipment. Misplacement, or rarely migration, of an epidural catheter into a blood vessel or the subarachnoid or subdural space may lead to serious problems. Local anaesthetic, opioid or combined infusions have the potential for different complications.

Complications associated with local anaesthetics

Epidural infusion
The most common side effect of epidural local anaesthetic is hypotension and this is more likely in the presence of hypovolaemia. Upright posture, density of block and high placement of the catheter in the thoracic epidural space may also lead to an increased incidence. Urinary retention may occur

in the presence of continuous epidural local anaesthetic blockade, but in the absence of sacral parasympathetic block this is not inevitable.[14, 15] The use of high concentrations of bupivacaine frequently leads to motor blockade in the lower limbs. This is unpleasant for the patient, limits postoperative mobility and risks the development of pressure sores.

Toxicity from prolonged infusion of bupivacaine is unlikely even when plasma concentrations are relatively high, and major problems should not occur suddenly in the absence of bolus administration.[7, 16] Postoperatively, the plasma concentration of alpha$_1$-acidglycoprotein, the protein which provides the main binding sites for bupivacaine increases. Total plasma concentrations of bupivacaine can therefore increase appreciably in the postoperative period without major alteration in free drug concentrations.[17]

Misplaced infusion

Accidental intravenous administration of bupivacaine may lead to central nervous system and cardiac toxicity, dependent on the absolute plasma concentration and its rate of increase.[18, 19] Cardiotoxicity due to bupivacaine in man occurs at a plasma concentration nearer to that which causes central nervous system toxicity than is the case with lignocaine.[20] Subarachnoid administration will lead to spinal anaesthesia. The rate of drug administration will determine the likelihood and speed of onset of total spinal block. Subdural administration will lead to a higher block than anticipated.[21]

Complications associated with opioids

Epidural infusion

Severe respiratory depression or apnoea is the most feared complication of epidural opioids. It is rare, but may occur without warning many hours after drug administration.[22] Late respiratory depression is more likely with morphine which is hydrophilic and ascends slowly within the cerebrospinal fluid.[23] Lipophilic opioids have a faster onset and a shorter duration which allows a continuous infusion to be more readily adapted to an individual patient's needs. Theoretically the risk of late respiratory depression would appear to be less when using a lipophilic opioid due to rapid clearance from the cerebrospinal fluid, but there have been recent reports of such late respiratory depression after fentanyl.[24, 25] It is known that fentanyl ascends to the cervical region in the cerebrospinal fluid within one hour of lumbar epidural administration and early respiratory depression may be secondary to systemic uptake or subarachnoid spread.[26, 27] Concurrent administration of systemic opioids increases the risk of respiratory depression.[28] There are no reports of respiratory depression when lipophilic drugs are given by epidural infusion only.

The fate of diamorphine after injection into the epidural space is not certain. It is stable in saline and bupivacaine solutions, is not metabolized to morphine in the cerebrospinal fluid and the rate of onset of analgesia and the plasma concentrations after its systemic uptake suggest that it remains as diamorphine in the epidural space.[29–32] However, the possibility that it is metabolized to morphine in epidural fat and subsequently crosses the dura cannot be excluded.

Pruritus and urinary retention are common side-effects of epidural opioids, but may be less common when infusions are used.[14] The incidence of nausea and vomiting associated with epidural opioids varies between studies, but may be less than with systemically administered opioids in some circumstances.[33–35]

Misplaced infusion
The only side effect of accidental intravenous infusion of epidural doses of opioid is less effective analgesia. Accidental subarachnoid administration is likely to increase the probability of respiratory depression, but has not been reported.

Management of the infusion

Successful management is dependent on reliable administrative procedures. These should ensure that an effective block is maintained and that there is early recognition of developing problems. The infusion technique may vary, but providing care is taken with the initial set up, nursing staff have clear guidelines and potential complications are considered in advance, a safe system can be devised. With such a system no single error should lead to a major complication.

Preparation

Care taken at this stage has a major influence on the subsequent safety of an epidural infusion.

Catheter insertion
The likelihood of catheter misplacement is reduced when it is sited preoperatively with the patient awake. The use of local anaesthetic blockade for the intraoperative phase helps to confirm correct placement and is recommended even when postoperative analgesia is to be provided using an epidural opioid alone. Single end-hole catheters may be safer than multiple side-hole catheters which can be sited with one orifice in the epidural space and another in the subarachnoid space or a vein, but they may lead to a higher incidence of unilateral blockade.[36]

Level of catheter insertion

The analgesia produced by a low dose epidural infusion is influenced by the level at which the catheter is sited. With a large bolus dose of local anaesthetic, an extensive block will be produced whether the catheter is sited in the lumbar or thoracic region. However, the block produced by the infusion of a small amount of drug is very dependent on the position of the catheter because it will gradually regress to encompass no more than a few dermatomes.[37] A low lumbar infusion is unlikely to maintain an adequate extent of block after abdominal surgery. This is the main, although perhaps not the only, factor explaining the tachyphylaxis described with postoperative epidural infusions.[38, 39] With opioids, the particular drug determines how much influence catheter site has on subsequent analgesia. Lumbar or caudal administration of morphine can prove very effective after abdominal or even thoracic surgery because slow clearance from the cerebrospinal fluid leads to more extensive spread in the subarachnoid space.[40–42] In contrast, lipophilic opioids are more effective when administered close to the dermatomal level of the operation.[43]

It is not possible to control where the catheter goes once it is within the epidural space and only 2–3 cm of an end-holed catheter should be inserted to ensure placement at the correct level.

Catheter fixation

It is important that the catheter is secured firmly to the patient's back when a continuous infusion is used. Patient movement and nursing care can easily dislodge an inadequately fixed catheter.

Filter

A bacterial filter should be attached at the time of catheter insertion and all solutions infused through it. A filter which allows aspiration without becoming damaged is preferable. If the infusion is prepared using drugs supplied in glass ampoules it is important to eliminate glass fragments from the solution. This may be achieved either by drawing the drug up through a particle filter or incorporating one (such as a blood filter) in the infusion line.

Initial block

A low dose epidural infusion of local anaesthetic will not produce good analgesia without the prior establishment of effective blockade using a suitable bolus dose of a long acting agent. In the lumbar region 10 ml of 0.5% bupivacaine administered within one hour of commencing the infusion is effective, but smaller doses are sufficient for thoracic block. It is wise to repeat the bolus dose immediately before the infusion is commenced if more than one hour has elapsed, or pain relief may prove inadequate in the early postoperative period. Problems after a bolus dose are usually apparent within twenty minutes at which time the patient will still be in theatre or the recovery room.

A bolus dose of epidural morphine may take an hour to be effective.[44] Lipophilic opioids have a faster onset, but *bolus* administration can lead to respiratory depression after one or two hours by which time the patient may have left the recovery room.[25] The provision of analgesia in the early postoperative period with epidural local anaesthetic and administration of opioids solely by infusion may avoid this complication.

Maintenance

Many techniques have been described for maintenance of analgesia using an epidural infusion.[7, 45, 46] The rate of administration of the solution may vary greatly. To some extent this reflects the siting of the catheter in relation to the site of surgery. A high thoracic infusion is usually given at a lower rate than a lumbar infusion to minimize side effects and also because the block is less likely to regress below the level of the wound after abdominal surgery. The effectiveness of epidural infusions is also dependent on the agents used. Local anaesthetics produce conduction blockade at nerve roots.[47] The number of dermatomes blocked is dependent on the spread of solution within the epidural space and this may be limited even when high volumes are used.[48] The infusion of a low volume of a low concentration of bupivacaine alone is ineffective although it may successfully improve analgesia provided by an opioid infusion.[13] In contrast, opioids act on receptors within the spinal cord.[49] The infusion of a low volume of a low concentration of an opioid can produce effective analgesia. This may be because within the cerebrospinal fluid the drug becomes more widely dispersed leading to more extensive blockade.[50] This is supported by the gradual rise in dermatomal block and the measurable levels of even lipophilic opioids within cervical cerebrospinal fluid after lumbar epidural administration.[26, 51]

It is useful to consider high and low volume epidural infusion techniques separately. Each method requires different equipment and the practical management varies. High volume infusions typically use rates of 10–25 ml.hour^{-1}. Low volume infusions may be given at rates of less than 1 ml.hour^{-1} but more commonly 2–5 ml.hour^{-1}.

High volume techniques

Large volumes of solution are unnecessary for effective use of epidural opioids and therefore almost invariably contain a local anaesthetic. This may be combined with an opioid for greater effect. Bupivacaine has been used in concentrations of 0.0625% to 1.0%, but the tendency is towards lower concentrations of drug.[14, 53] This may reduce the total dose of bupivacaine administered, but doses of less than 15 mg. hour^{-1} are

seldom effective alone whatever volume or concentration is employed.[48]
It has been shown that analgesia, extent of sensory block and side effects
such as motor blockade are dependent more on the total dose of drug
than on concentration or volume of the solution, and the necessity for
high volume local anaesthetic infusions must be questioned. However,
there may be safety advantages associated with their use and this will
be discussed later in this chapter. It is still important to site the catheter
carefully having regard to the dermatomes requiring blockade.

Low volume techniques
Low volume techniques are usually based on the use of opioids. Combinations of drugs may again prove superior and the addition of doses of
bupivacaine that are ineffective alone can improve analgesia.[13]

Administering a high volume infusion
Solutions containing low concentrations of bupivacaine are not available
commercially and have to be prepared by diluting ampoules of more
concentrated drug. A standard method of preparation with as few steps
as possible reduces the possibility of error and the time involved. The
necessity to prepare the solution using intravenous fluid bags means
that great care must be taken to ensure that the solution is not given
intravenously in error.

1. The contents should be labelled by writing on the bag with an
indelible marker as well as with an additive label.
2. The bag should be connected to the epidural system immediately
after preparation by the anaesthetist responsible for the infusion. Tubing
with Luer locks is advisable to prevent disconnection and labelling of the
tubing will provide added safety, especially in patients with multiple
infusion lines.
3. The preparation of sufficient solution for the duration of the infusion
eliminates the possibility of error during the changing of bags.

The addition of 10 ampoules of 10 ml 0.75% bupivacaine plain solution
to a 500 ml bag of 0.9% saline produces 600 ml of 0.125% bupivacaine,
sufficient for 40 hours at 15 ml.hour^{-1}. Using 10 ml ampoules of 0.5%
bupivacaine will give 600 ml of a 0.083% solution. The addition
of diamorphine 20mg allows the administration of 0.5 mg. hour^{-1}
of diamorphine at 15 ml.hour^{-1}. This reservoir of solution contains
potentially lethal doses of drugs, so that the system used for its delivery
must be failsafe. An advantage of a high volume system is that the patient
may be connected directly to only an aliquot of this solution. The main
reservoir is isolated from the patient except during replenishment of an
intermediate container. With this system no single error can result in the
patient receiving a very large dose of drug.

A volumetric pump can be used as shown in Fig. 7.1. A burette is situated between the reservoir and the pump. The tap between the reservoir and the burette is only opened to allow refilling of the burette and is then immediately closed. In the event of rapid administration of epidural solution due to pump malfunction or incorrect setting, the patient can only receive the contents of the burette. The maximum volume in the burette should be safe for bolus administration; the volume infused over a 2-hour period is usually a safe maximum. Nursing staff must understand the need for the burette and the danger of circumventing it by leaving the connection from the reservoir open. The ideal burette has a capacity equal to the refill volume and cannot be overfilled. Paediatric burettes with a volume of 30 ml are readily available (Avon Medical). When a larger burette is used the maximum volume permitted in the burette should be carefully specified.

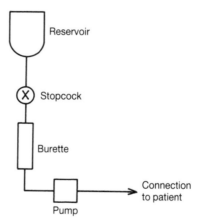

Figure 7.1 Set up for administering a high volume epidural infusion using a volumetric pump.

A syringe driver may be used for high volume epidural infusions using a closed system as shown in Fig. 7.2. The safety of this system is dependent on the use of an appropriate three-way connection which allows the reservoir to be connected to the syringe or the syringe to the patient, but does not permit connection of the reservoir to the patient or all three channels to be open at the same time. A device such as the antishunt stopcock with additional double female Luer adaptor (Medex Medical Inc.) is suitable. The syringe may be safely refilled at 2-hourly intervals by nursing staff with no possibility of error. The danger of additional gravity feed from the reservoir into the patient during the infusion is also eliminated.

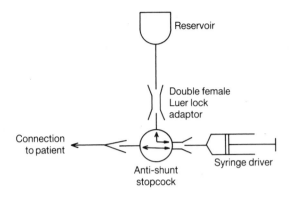

Reservoir

Double female
Luer lock
adaptor

Connection
to patient

Syringe driver

Anti-shunt
stopcock

Figure 7.2 Set up for administering a high volume epidural infusion using a syringe driver.

Administering a low volume infusion

A low volume epidural infusion may be administered with a syringe driver using a 10 or 20 ml syringe. This system is often used for opioids alone. It may be set up rapidly and is portable and cheap. It is capable of accidental connection to an intravenous cannula, but a more important disadvantage is that the patient is connected directly to a potentially lethal dose of drug and the safety of the method is very dependent on reliable pump function. Paediatric volumetric cartridge pumps, although less portable, also allow accurate low volume administration. When rates of the order of 5 ml.hour^{-1} are employed a burette may be used with such a pump, or the syringe driver system as described for high volume infusions may be used. Below this volume the rate of administration is so small that these systems are impractical and there is then no fail safe capability.

Assessments

The continued safety and comfort of the patient after surgery is very dependent on good nursing care. Nurses perform frequent postoperative assessments, record their observations and, in the event of a problem, provide first line management. Nursing observation may be supplemented by the use of cardiorespiratory monitoring equipment appropriate to the patient and the clinical situation. Further postoperative assessment should be provided by the anaesthetic staff and, on occasion, the patient.

Nursing assessment

Postoperative epidural infusions can cause concern in nurses who have no experience of them and it is less than ideal if the technique is used on an occasional basis. When the technique is introduced on a ward where the staff are unfamiliar with its use it is essential that anaesthetic staff are readily available to answer queries and educate the nurses. Smooth and safe conduct of epidural infusion analgesia is achieved if nursing staff are aware of the potential problems, know how to avoid them and know how to deal with any difficulties that may arise. A helpful aid is the provision of a chart which clearly sets out the patient observations required, notes the prescription of the infusion and details appropriate action for potential problems. Such clearly established guidelines, coupled with the ready availability of a designated anaesthetist, will usually lead to rapid nursing acceptance of the technique especially once the superior pain relief is witnessed.

Patient observations

Many of these observations will be performed after surgery, no matter what type of analgesic regimen is used, but the frequency or duration of such recordings may need to be modified while the epidural infusion is in progress. Some observations are more applicable to the use of epidural local anaesthetic than epidural opioid and vice versa.

1. *Pulse and blood pressure.* It is prudent to make recordings every 15 minutes for the first 2 hours postoperatively, then at increasing, but regular, intervals providing the patient is stable. If a bolus dose of local anaesthetic is required continuous nursing observation is recommended and recordings should be made at 5 minute intervals for 20–30 minutes. In the absence of hypovolaemia blood pressure is usually well maintained in the conscious patient with an epidural block. However, even a minor degree of hypovolaemia may produce marked hypotension *without* compensatory tachycardia. Blood loss may be concealed internally or considerable losses of circulating volume may follow major surgery (e.g. aortic reconstruction) and this should be considered.

A patient with pink feet and cold blue hands may be compensating with marked upper limb vasoconstriction for a lack of circulating volume in the presence of lower limb sympathetic blockade. This is a classical sign, but it should be stressed that the presence of warm, pink hands does not necessarily mean that all is well, because a very high sympathetic block may be present. With such a high block significant hypovolaemia may be expected to lead to profound hypotension requiring urgent treatment.

2. *Respiratory rate.* This is an extremely crude measure of the effects of epidural opioids on respiration. Apnoea occurring without previous depression of respiratory rate has been described, as has severe ventilatory depression in the presence of a normal respiratory rate. [8, 22] Despite this, slowing of respiration in the presence of an epidural opioid infusion may forewarn of the possibility of more severe respiratory depression.

3. *Level of sedation.* It has been suggested that somnolence may be a more relevant warning of impending respiratory depression.[8] It may be that

in such patients some respiratory depression has already occurred and that the decreased conscious level is a reflection of CO_2 retention, although this has not been documented.

4. *Height of block.* It is not our routine practice to expect nurses to check the height of the block to pinprick or ice, but rather to encourage them to obtain anaesthetic assistance should they be concerned about the patient's vital signs. However, experienced nurses may wish to check on the height of the block at intervals to reassure themselves that all is well. Such interest should be encouraged, but not at the expense of the patient's sleep pattern.

5. *Motor power.* An assessment of the degree of weakness in the legs should be made at intervals. Increasing intensity of motor blockade may indicate intrathecal infusion of local anaesthetic and should be reported. It may also be a consequence of excessive epidural block and in these cases it is important that skin damage is prevented by pressure care. Any evidence of increasing weakness of upper or lower limbs demands assessment by medical staff.

6. *Urine output.* There is conflicting evidence about the incidence of urinary retention during epidural infusions of local anaesthetics or opioids.[44, 54] There is no doubt that urinary retention is more frequent when a combination of drugs is administered[12] and it is important not to allow bladder distension in patients who do not have an indwelling catheter. This can easily be prevented if proper recordings are made and should be considered if non-specific abdominal discomfort occurs. If the patient is catheterized urine output can provide useful information about the adequacy of the circulation.

7. *Degree of analgesia.* Most monitoring is directed at the identification and prevention of complications of surgery or the block. However it is important that nurses check the adequacy of pain relief by direct questioning. Clear instructions on dealing with inadequate pain relief should be available and this is discussed later.

Management and recording of infusion volumes.
The volume of solution infused must be recorded at least hourly by direct observation of the contents of the burette or syringe.

Anaesthetic assessment

An anaesthetist must be available in the hospital to respond to acute problems at all times when an epidural infusion is in progress. The overall management of the patient remains the responsibility of the anaesthetist instituting the block. The first requirement is the establishment of adequate analgesia in the immediate postoperative period. Early assessment and recording of the height of block to pinprick establishes a baseline for subsequent comparisons during the course of the infusion. If block height is determined once the patient is fully conscious, an ascending block can be picked up at an early stage and managed appropriately. An occasional assessment by a member of the medical staff will confirm that the infusion is progressing safely. This should include a review of the nursing observations.

Patient self-assessment

The patient should be asked to report any untoward effects during the infusion, in particular, increasing spread of numbness, or weakness of lower or upper limbs.

Monitoring equipment

The use of epidural infusions outwith intensive care or high dependency areas remains controversial and some would suggest that safety may be increased by the instrumental monitoring of patients.[55] Pulse oximetry is a simple, non-invasive method of monitoring which will readily identify episodes of desaturation. However, in practice it may be difficult to obtain a reliable signal from a conscious patient and concurrent oxygen therapy may obscure the presence of hypoventilation. Measurement of the expired carbon dioxide concentration may detect hypoventilation, but is even less convenient to use in the postoperative patient on a general ward. Inductance plethysmography has a number of theoretical attractions, but is largely a research technique at present.

Management of complications

The safety of the patient must be the first consideration when using an epidural infusion. In common with all medical procedures, the likelihood of major problems is reduced when patients are managed by experienced staff who have written guidelines immediately available. It should not be assumed that junior medical staff have the knowledge or ability to manage significant side-effects and they too should have clear instructions on immediate management especially when to seek senior advice.

Inadequate analgesia

No technique is 100% successful in all patients and it is important to deal with inadequate analgesia promptly and effectively. Too often patients are provided with meagre reassurance rather than positive action to relieve pain. The appropriate management depends on the clinical environment, the drugs already being infused and, to some extent, on the time at which pain relief becomes insufficient (Table 7.1).

In the recovery area

Immediately after surgery it is essential that the patient is comfortable with an adequately functioning epidural block, because the infusion by itself will not establish analgesia. If there is a problem with the epidural at this stage it is better to replace the catheter sooner rather than later and adequate pain relief can be provided quickly. With some types of surgery this option may not be practical, e.g. after aortic reconstruction with the administration of anticoagulants. Visceral pain may be a source of discomfort even in the presence of a full somatic block of the wound. This responds readily to small doses of systemic opioid which may be given intravenously at this time. If it is planned to administer epidural opioids subsequently, monitoring in a high dependency situation would then be mandatory.

Later in the postoperative period

By this time the effect of the bolus dose of local anaesthetic given in the theatre or the recovery room is regressing. Usually the early institution of the infusion will prevent the development of pain, but it may occur in some patients. The correct course of action will depend on the type of epidural infusion being employed. When a local anaesthetic is infused and a somatic block is still evident many patients benefit from the administration of an intramuscular opioid. Severe pain implies that the block has regressed significantly and a bolus dose of bupivacaine may be required. However, other causes of the patient's pain should be considered. These include complications of surgery, urinary retention or displacement of the epidural catheter. A clear feature of intravenous migration of the catheter is complete loss of evidence of somatic block. The dose of bupivacaine administered by epidural infusion is unlikely to lead to features of systemic toxicity when infused intravenously, but a subsequent bolus dose may produce severe toxic effects. The patient's cardiovascular status should be considered before a bolus is administered.

If analgesia is inadequate when infusing an epidural opioid alone a bolus of local anaesthetic may be very effective. If pain relief again becomes inadequate the addition of a low dose of local anaesthetic to the opioid infusion should be considered. Even very small amounts of bupivacaine (2–4 mg.hour^{-1}) can prove effective in this situation, but should be preceded by a further bolus dose of local anaesthetic. Individual requirements for epidural opioids vary widely and a bolus

Table 7.1   Management of inadequate analgesia

Recovery room

1.   Ensure local anaesthetic block is adequate:

(a)   Bolus dose of 0.5% bupivacaine within one hour of commencing infusion.
(b)   Replace catheter if problem achieving an acceptable block.

2.   If analgesia remains inadequate despite good somatic block:

(a) Consider likelihood of problems, e.g., bladder distension.
(b) Administer increments of opioid intravenously. If an epidural infusion of opioid alone or in combination has been used, high dependency care is considered mandatory.

Later in the postoperative period	
Type of infusion	Action

Local anaesthetic alone

No somatic block	Check catheter and pump. If no problem identified, either replace catheter or give very cautious bolus dose of local anaesthetic.
Poor somatic block	Check catheter and pump. Give very cautious dose of local anaesthetic.
Good somatic block	Give intravenous or intramuscular opioid.

Opioid alone

Reinstate block with local anaesthetic. If this results in:

Good somatic block	If analgesia becomes inadequate again give further dose of local anaesthetic and switch to combined infusion.
No somatic block	Resite epidural catheter or switch to intramuscular opioid.

Combined local anaesthetic and opioid infusion

No somatic block	Check catheter and pump. If no problem identified, either replace catheter or give very cautious dose of local anaesthetic.
Poor somatic block	Check catheter and pump. Give very cautious dose of local anaesthetic
Good somatic block	Very careful consideration of other reasons for pain. A bolus dose of opioid by any route makes high dependency care mandatory.

dose of opioid given epidurally may resolve the problem, but, as with additional systemic administration of opioids, this makes high dependency care mandatory.[3]

Inadequate analgesia when using a combined local anaesthetic and opioid infusion is less frequent than with a single agent. If it is clear that the infusion is still being delivered to the epidural space, but further analgesia is required, a small bolus dose of local anaesthetic should be effective.

Masking of postoperative complications

The use of epidural infusions should not cause difficulty with the diagnosis of postoperative complications *provided the surgical staff are aware that effective analgesia may modify the presenting features*. In particular, there may be a tendency to ascribe hypotension to the effects of epidural blockade rather than blood loss. Bladder distension may lead to breakthrough pain and should always be considered in patients without a urinary catheter.

Hypotension

Hypotension is more likely in the immediate postoperative period after the administration of relatively large doses of local anaesthetic in theatre. It occurs less commonly in the later postoperative course when a stable level of block is maintained by an infusion.

Prevention
Prompt replacement of intraoperative blood loss with appropriate fluid is essential to maintain circulating volume. The routine use of large volumes of crystalloid in an effort to reduce the incidence of hypotension is misguided. It is ineffective and an increased incidence of urinary retention may be expected.[56] Left ventricular failure may be precipitated in patients with poor myocardial function as the sympathetic block regresses.

Intramuscular ephedrine (30 mg) given at the end of surgery is effective in reducing the incidence of hypotension without causing significant adverse cardiovascular changes.[57]

Treatment
The initial management of postoperative hypotension is not affected by the presence of an epidural block. The patient should be given oxygen by facemask and the lower limbs elevated to improve venous return.This will not affect the height of the block. If hypotension persists 250 ml of 0.9% saline should be given intravenously as rapidly as possible and the responsible anaesthetist informed. When these simple methods fail to maintain blood pressure, careful consideration should be given to the

possibilities of haemorrhage or extension of the block: in either case 30 mg of ephedrine may be given intramuscularly to support the circulation whilst these are being investigated.

Further assessment should include careful assessment of blood volume and evidence for continued fluid or blood loss. If concealed blood loss remains a possibility after treatment of a hypotensive episode the frequency of nursing observations should be increased. The height of the block should be determined and compared with previous recordings. It is unusual for a block to extend further cephalad once the infusion has been in progress for 2–3 hours. If a sensory block extends gradually the infusion should be stopped for a period of time and consideration should be given to the possibility of catheter migration, especially if motor block in the legs increases as well. The height of the block should be determined more frequently thereafter.

Respiratory depression

The controversial question of the use of epidural opioids in patients in a general ward is considered in Chapter 10 and the factors which influence the risk in Chapter 6.

Prevention
At present it would appear that the safest technique is a constant low dose infusion of a lipophilic drug and the avoidance of large bolus doses.

Treatment
Respiratory depression due to epidural opioids responds to intravenous naloxone, which may need to be given repeatedly or by infusion. Analgesia may not be significantly impaired after naloxone when epidural bupivacaine is also being administered or the opioid in question is morphine. With lipophilic drugs such as fentanyl sufficient naloxone to reverse respiratory depression antagonizes analgesia.[58, 59]

Urinary retention

Epidural opioids and local anaesthetics may lead to an increased incidence of postoperative urinary retention especially when the drugs are administered together.[12] Many patients will require bladder catheterization for surgical indications or accurate monitoring of urine output. If the patient is unable to void spontaneously, intravenous naloxone may allow micturition and should be given in 0.1 mg increments every 2–3 minutes up to 0.4 mg. If this is ineffective bladder catheterization should be performed and occasionally may need to be repeated.[8]

Pruritus

This is a frequent side effect of epidural opioids, but is usually trivial and does not distress the patient or require treatment. It is important to explain to the patient, the nursing and junior medical staff that the symptom is caused by the epidural infusion and will not respond to creams or antihistaminics. The occasional patient who has troublesome pruritus should receive intravenous naloxone.[59] A single dose of 0.4 mg is often sufficient. Intramuscular doses of naloxone 0.4 mg may be given as required by nursing staff if the symptom recurs.

Nausea and vomiting

Epidural opioids are associated with nausea and vomiting which may respond to antiemetics. Naloxone may be tried for intractable vomiting especially when a combined local anaesthetic and opioid infusion is in progress.[60]

Difficulty with mobilization

Epidural opioid infusions permit easy patient mobilization because of the absence of sympathetic and motor blockade and the use of small portable syringe drivers.

The use of epidural bupivacaine does not preclude patient mobilization, but problems may be encountered. Young, fit patients can normally be mobilized progressively and even walk around with a demonstrable thoracic sensory block. Older patients may not be able to compensate so readily and greater care must be exercised. Ease of mobilization is probably related to the use of very low doses of bupivacaine. In some patients motor blockade makes mobilization difficult and in these cases the epidural infusion may be converted to opioid alone or discontinued.

Epidural catheter problems

A major advantage of epidural infusion techniques compared to bolus administration is that the effects of catheter migration into the subarachnoid space or a blood vessel are gradual rather than sudden. An awareness of these possibilities and the presenting features is essential.

Subarachnoid infusion
The clinical effects of continuous infusion of high volumes of dilute local anaesthetic solutions into the subarachnoid space have not been

established. It is likely that even at 20 ml. hour^{-1} total spinal anaesthesia will take many minutes, if not hours to occur, but it is important not to dismiss the possibility.[61] An unusually dense block or one which has extended significantly should be viewed with suspicion, especially if associated with profound or re-established motor blockade. A careful aspiration test should be performed and if there is any doubt the safest course of action is to replace the catheter.

Intrathecal migration when opioids alone are being administered may result in severe respiratory depression. Local anaesthetic used in combination with an opioid may reveal at an earlier stage that this complication has occurred.

Intravenous infusion

The doses of drugs administered by epidural infusion are unlikely to cause any systemic symptoms even after many hours of intravenous infusion. The most likely result will be diminution in analgesia and loss of a demonstrable block. Toxic effects will occur if a rapid bolus of drug is given in an attempt to re-establish analgesia. A careful aspiration test and slow administration of any such dose is imperative.

Problems specific to the type of surgery

Management of an epidural infusion may require modification as a consequence of the type of surgery performed. When intraoperative anticoagulation with heparin has taken place during major vascular surgery, the decision to replace a displaced catheter in the immediate postoperative period must be taken with care because there may be an increased risk of epidural haematoma formation. Some orthopaedic surgeons may view the possibility of urinary catheterization with dismay in case transient bacteraemia leads to infection after major joint replacement. The use of bupivacaine or an opioid alone may be preferable to the combination. Naloxone will be more effective when only an opioid has been given. If bupivacaine alone has been used the infusion may be allowed to wear off fairly quickly if necessary. Specific situations such as these demand careful thought and management policies that have been agreed with the surgeon in advance.

Discontinuing the infusion

The epidural infusion may be discontinued after a specified period of time dependent on the operation performed and the availability of postoperative care and equipment. The continued comfort of the patient should be considered when this is done and it is illogical to devote a great deal of effort for an arbitrary period of time if the patient then only recollects the late onset of severe pain.

Conclusion

Continuous epidural infusion of local anaesthetic and opioid drugs can provide postoperative analgesia unsurpassed by any other technique. These methods should be part of the armamentarium available for pain relief after major surgery.

Acceptance of this is dependent on good medical practice. It is a simple matter to set up an epidural infusion. Its safe and optimal use requires commitment, education, planning and common sense.

References

1.   Dawkins M. Relief of postoperative pain by continuous epidural drip. *Surv. Anesthesiol.* 1957; **1**: 616–7.
2.   Gambling D. R., Yu P., Cole C., McMorland G. H., Palmer L. A comparative study of patient controlled epidural analgesia (PCEA) and continuous infusion epidural analgesia (CIEA) during labour. *Can. J. Anaesth.* 1988; **35**: 249–54.
3.   Sjostrom S., Hartvig D., Tamsen A. Patient-controlled analgesia with extradural morphine or pethidine. *Brit. J. Anaesth.* 1988; **60**: 358–66.
4.   Kalia P. K., Madan R., Batra R. K., Latha V., Vardham V., Gode, G. R. Clinical study on epidural clonidine for postoperative analgesia. *Ind. J. Med. Res.* 1986; **83**: 550–2
5.   Naguib, M., Adu-Gyamfi Y., Absood G. H., Farag H., Gyasi H. K. Epidural ketamine for postoperative analgesia. *Can. Anaesth. Soc. J.* 1986; **33**: 16–21.
6.   Tucker G. T. Pharmacokinetics of local anaesthetics. *Brit. J. Anaesth.* 1986; **58**: 717–31.
7.   Ross R. A., Clarke J. E., Armitage E. N. Postoperative pain prevention by continuous epidural infusion. A study of the clinical effects and the plasma concentrations obtained. *Anaesthesia* 1980; **35**: 663–8.
8.   Ready L. B., Oden R., Chadwick H. S., Benedetti C., Rooke G. A., Caplan R., Wild L. M. Development of an anesthesiology-based postoperative pain management service. *Anesthesiology.* 1988; **68**: 100–6.
9.   Torda T. A., Pybus D. A. Comparison of four narcotic analgesics for extradural analgesia. *Brit. J. Anaesth.* 1982; **54**: 291–5.
10. Simpson K. J. H., Madej T. H., McDowell J. M., MacDonald R., Lyons G. Comparison of extradural buprenorphine and extradural morphine after caesarean section. *Brit. J. Anaesth.* 1988; **60**: 627–31.
11. Lippmann M., Mok. M. S. Epidural butorphanol for the relief of postoperative pain. *Anesthesia and Analgesia* 1988; **67**: 418–21.
12. Lee A., Simpson D., Whitfield A., Scott D. B. Postoperative analgesia by continuous extradural infusion of bupivacaine and diamorphine. *Brit. J. Anaesth.* 1988; **60**: 845–50.

13. Cullen M. L., Staren E. D., El-Ganzouri A., Logas W. G., Ivankovich, A. D., Economou S. G. Continuous epidural infusion for analgesia after major abdominal operations: a randomized, prospective, double-blind study. *Surg.* 1985; **98**: 718–26.

14. El-Baz N. M. L., Faber L. P., Jensik R. J. Continuous epidural infusion of morphine for treatment of pain after thoracic surgery: a new technique. *Anesthesia and Analgesia* 1984; **63**: 757–64.

15. Cousins M. J., Bromage P. R. Epidural neural blockade. In: *Neural Blockade in Clinical Anesthesia and Management of Pain. (edn. 2)* Philadelphia, J. B. Lippincott Co. 1988.

16. Rosenblatt R., Pepitone-Rockwell F., McKillop M. J. Continuous axillary analgesia for traumatic hand injury. *Anesthesiology.* 1979; **51**: 565–6.

17. Wulf H., Winckler K., Maier C. H., Heinzow B. Pharmacokinetics and protein binding of bupivacaine in postoperative epidural analgesia. *Acta Anaesthesiol. Scand.* 1988; **32**: 530–4.

18. Jorfeldt L., Lofstrom B., Pernow B., Persson B., Wahren J., Widman, B. The effect of local anaesthetics on the central circulation and respiration in man and dog. *Acta Anaesthesiol. Scand.* 1968; **12**: 153–69.

19. Scott D. B. Evaluation of the toxicity of local anaesthetic agents in man. *Brit. J. Anaesth.* 1975; **47**: 56–61.

20. Reiz S., Math S. Cardiotoxicity of local anaesthetic agents. *Brit. J. Anaesth.* 1986; **58**: 736–46.

21. Lee A., Dodd K. W. Accidental subdural catheterization. *Anaesthesia* 1986; **41**: 847–9.

22. Wust H. J., Bromage P. R. Delayed respiratory arrest after epidural hydromorphone. *Anaesthesia* 1987; **42**: 404-406.

23. Gourlay G. K., Cherry D. A., Cousins M. J. Cephalad migration of morphine in CSF following lumbar epidural administration in patients with cancer pain. *Pain* 1985; **23**: 317–26.

24. Wells D. G., Davies G. Profound central nervous system depression from epidural fentanyl for extracorporeal shock wave lithotripsy. *Anaesthesiology* 1987; **67**: 991–2.

25. Brockway M. S., Noble D. W., Sharwood-Smith G. H., McClure J. H. Profound respiratory depression after extradural fentanyl. *Brit. J. Anaesth.* 1990;**64:** 243–5.

26. Gourlay G. K., Murphy T. M., Plummer J. L., Kowalski S. R., Cherry D. A., Cousins M. J. Pharmacokinetics of fentanyl in lumbar and cervical CSF following lumbar epidural and intravenous administration. *Pain* 1989; **38**: 253–9.

27. Ahuja B. R., Strunin L. Respiratory effects of epidural fentanyl. Changes in end-tidal CO_2 and respiratory rate following single doses and continuous infusions of epidural fentanyl. *Anaesthesia* 1985; **40**: 949–55.

28. Scott D. B., McClure J. Selective epidural analgesia. *Lancet* 1979; **1**: 1410–1.

29. Hanks G. W., Hoskin P. J., Walker V. A. Diamorphine stability and pharmacodynamics. *Anaesthesia* 1987; **42**: 664–5.

30. Moore A., Bullingham R., McQuay H., Allen M., Baldwin D., Cole A. Spinal fluid kinetics of morphine and heroin. *Clin. Pharmacol. Ther.* 1984; **35**: 40–5.

31. Watson J., Moore A., McQuay H., Teddy P., Baldwin D., Allen M., Bullingham R. Plasma morphine concentrations and analgesic effects of

lumbar extradural morphine and heroin. *Anesthesia and Analgesia* 1984; **63**: 629–34.

32. Jacobson L., Phillips P. S., Hull C. J., Conacher I. D. Extradural versus intramuscular diamorphine. A controlled study of analgesic and adverse effects in the postoperative period. *Anaesthesia* 1983; **38**: 10–8.

33. Eisenach J. C., Grice S. C., Dewan D. M. Patient-controlled analgesia following cesarean section: a comparison with epidural and intramuscular narcotics. *Anesthesiology* 1988; **68**: 444–8.

34. Pybus D. A., Torda T. A. Dose-effect relationships of extradural morphine. *Brit. J. Anaesth.* 1982; **54**: 1259–62.

35. Harrison D. M., Sinatra R., Morgese L., Chung J. H. Epidural narcotic and patient-controlled analgesia for post-cesarean section pain relief. *Anesthesiology.* 1988; **68**: 454–7.

36. Scott D. B. Test doses in extradural block. *Brit. J. Anaesth.* 1988; **61**: 129–30.

37. Raj P. P., Knarr D. C., Vigdorth E., Denson D. D., Pither C. E., Hartrick C. T., Hopson C. N., Edstrom H. Comparison of continuous epidural infusion of a local anesthetic and administration of systemic narcotics in the management of pain after total knee replacement surgery. *Anesthesia and Analgesia* 1987; **66**: 401–6.

38. Mogensen T., Hjortso N. C., Bigler D., Lund C., Kehlet H. Unpredictability of regression of analgesia during the continuous postoperative extradural infusion of bupivacaine. *Brit. J. Anaesth.* 1988; **60**: 515–9.

39. Mogensen T., Hojgaard L., Scott N. B., Henriksen J. H., Kehlet H. Epidural blood flow and regression of sensory analgesia during continuous postoperative epidural infusion of bupivacaine. *Anesthesia and Analgesia* 1988; **67**: 809–13.

40. Planner R. S., Cowie R. W., Babarczy A. S. Continuous epidural morphine analgesia after radical operations upon the pelvis. *Surg., Gynecol. Obst.* 1988; **166**: 229–32.

41. Rosen K. R., Rosen D. A. Caudal epidural morphine for control of pain following open heart surgery in children. *Anesthesiology.* 1989; **70**: 418–21.

42. Sjostrom S., Hartvig P., Persson P., Tamsen A. Pharmacokinetics of epidural morphine and meperidine in humans. *Anesthesiology* 1987; **67**: 877–88.

43. Mackersie R. C., Shackford S. R., Hoyt D. B., Karagianes T. G. Continuous epidural fentanyl analgesia: ventilatory function improvement with routine use in treatment of blunt chest injury. *J. Trauma* 1987; **27**: 1207–10.

44. Weddel S. J., Ritter R. R. Serum levels following epidural administration of morphine and correlation with relief of postsurgical pain. *Anesthesiology* 1981; **54**: 210–4.

45. Bailey P. W., Smith B. E. Continuous epidural infusion of fentanyl for postoperative analgesia. *Anaesthesia* 1980; **35**: 1002–6

46. Logas W. G., El-Baz N., El-Ganzouri A., Cullen M., Staren E., Faber P., Ivankovich A. D. Continuous thoracic epidural analgesia for postoperative pain relief following thoracotomy: a randomized prospective study. *Anesthesiology* 1987; **67**: 787–91.

47. Cousins M. J., Mather L. E. Intrathecal and epidural administration of opioids. *Anesthesiology* 1984; **61**: 276–310.

48. Lee A., Brockway M., McKeown D., Wildsmith J. A. W. Comparison of high and low volume extradural infusions for postoperative analgesia. (unpublished observations).
49. Atweh S. F., Kuhar M. J. Autoradiographic localization of opiate receptors in rat brain. I. Spinal cord and lower medulla. *Brain Res.* 1977; **124**: 53–67.
50. Gourlay G. K., Cherry D. A., Plummer J. L., Armstrong P. J., Cousins M. J. Influence of drug polarity on the absorption of opioid drugs into CSF and subsequent cephalad migration following lumbar epidural administration: application to morphine and pethidine. *Pain* 1987; **31**: 297–305.
51. Bromage P. R., Camporesi E. M., Durant P. A. C., Nielsen C. H. Rostral spread of epidural morphine. *Anesthesiology* 1982; **56**: 431–6.
52. Fischer R. L., Lubenow T. R., Liceaga A., McCarthy R. J., Ivankovich A. D. Comparison of continuous epidural infusion of fentanyl–bupivacaine and morphine–bupivacaine in management of postoperative pain. *Anesthesia and Analgesia* 1988; **67**: 559–63.
53. Renck H., Edstrom H., Kinnberger B., Brandt G. Thoracic epidural analgesia-II: prolongation in the early postoperative period by continuous injection of 1.0% bupivacaine. *Acta Anaesth. Scand.* 1976; **20**: 47–56.
54. Reiz S., Ahlin J., Ahrenfeldt B., Andersson M., Andersson S. Epidural morphine for postoperative pain relief. *Acta Anaesth. Scand.* 1981; **25**: 111–4.
55. Etches R. C., Sandler A. N., Daley M. D. Respiratory depression and spinal opioids. *Can. J. Anaesth.* 1989; **36**: 165–85.
56. Coe A. J., Revanas B. Is crystalloid preloading useful in spinal anaesthesia in the elderly. *Anaesthesia* 1990; **45**: 241–3.
57. Bowler G. M. R., Scott D. B. Segmental blockade and systolic pressure during overnight continuous infusion of 0.1 or 0.125% bupivacaine. *Vth Congress Eur. Soc. Reg. Anaesth.* Malmo, Sweden. 1986: 22.
58. Gueneron J. P., Ecoffey C., Carli P., Bvenhamou D., Gross J. B. Effect of naloxone infusion on analgesia and respiratory depression after epidural fentanyl. *Anesthesia and Analgesia* 1988; **67**: 35–8.
59. Korbon G. A., James D. J., Verlander J. M., Difazio C. A., Rosenblum S. M., Levy S. J., Perry P. C. Intramuscular naloxone reverses the side effects of epidural morphine while preserving analgesia. *Reg. Anesthesia* 1985; **10**: 16–20.
60. Rawal N., Schott U., Dahlstrom B., Intunisi C. E., Tandon B., Sjostrand V., Wennhager M. Influence of naloxone infusion on analgesia and respiratory depression following epidural morphine. *Anesthesiology* 1986; **64**: 194–201.
61. Evans T. I. Total spinal anaesthesia. *Anaesth. and Int. Care* 1974; **2**: 158–63.

8

Thoracic Nerve Block

A. Mowbray

Introduction

Local anaesthetic techniques can be of immense benefit to patients after abdominal and thoracic surgery. The adverse sequelae of these surgical procedures are well documented as are the beneficial effects on metabolism of local blocks. Whilst good analgesia may not be reflected in a major improvement in respiratory function this must not detract from the general improvement in the patient's well-being. Many anaesthetists feel that central blocks are relatively contraindicated in this branch of surgery because of autonomic side-effects and for this reason they look to more distal injections. However, it must be remembered that life-threatening complications may also be associated with these distal techniques. While single injections of long-acting local anaesthetic agents can be repeated as often as necessary to provide postoperative analgesia, it is undoubtedly more efficient, quicker and kinder to use a catheter technique if possible. By such methods appropriate and effective pain relief can be continued until oral analgesic drugs are sufficient. We must also guard against the belief that if a patient has a properly functioning block he will not require additional analgesia; apart from the fact that somatic pain may not always follow the accepted anatomical pathways, visceral pain may be unaffected by peripheral thoracic blocks.

Anatomy

In the thoracic region twelve pairs of nerves emerge from the spinal medulla and leave the vertebral canal through the intervertebral foramina. Each spinal nerve is attached to the medulla by a dorsal sensory and a ventral motor root with the sleeves of dura mater covering the roots becoming continuous with the epineurium of the spinal nerves. The ventral roots contain large myelinated fibres which supply the striated muscles of the body wall, and fine myelinated fibres of two types: motor to the intrafusal muscle spindles and preganglionic sympathetic fibres. These traverse the ventral root and emerge from it in the white ramus communicans, to enter the corresponding sympathetic ganglion. The dorsal roots contain sensory nerve fibres of all diameters, both myelinated and unmyelinated.

As the spinal nerve emerges from the intervertebral foramen it enters the paravertebral space, gives off a meningeal branch and divides into dorsal and ventral rami, both of which contain motor and sensory fibres. The paravertebral space is wedge-shaped, the base being formed by the posterolateral aspect of the body of the vertebra, and the intervertebral foramen and its contents.[1] Anteriorly lies the parietal pleura and posteriorly, the superior costo-transverse ligament, running from the lower border of the transverse process above, to the upper border of the rib below. The paravertebral space is bounded above and below by the heads and necks of adjacent ribs. Medially, it connects with the epidural space through the intervertebral foramen, and lateral to the tip of the transverse process it is continuous with the intercostal space (Fig. 8.1).

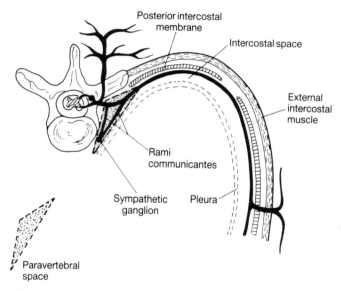

Figure 8.1 Diagramatic representation of the continuity of the paravertebral and intercostal spaces.

The dorsal rami in the thoracic region supply the erector spinae muscles and the skin, fascia, ligaments, bones and joints of the posterior part of the trunk. The ventral rami are mainly distributed to the lateral and anterior aspects of the trunk and are joined near their origin by a delicate bundle of non-myelinated, postganglionic fibres from the sympathetic trunk (grey ramus communicans). These fibres are distributed to blood vessels and sweat glands in the territory of the nerve they enter. In the thoracic region the twelve ventral rami are distributed in a regular segmental manner emerging inferior to the corresponding vertebrae and rib. The rostral eleven nerves are intercostal in position while the twelfth lies below the associated rib and is therefore the subcostal nerve.

A typical thoracic ventral ramus is thus connected to the sympathetic trunk by a grey and a white ramus communicans and sweeps forwards in the upper part of the intercostal space, frequently sending a collateral branch along the lower part of the same space.

The intercostal space lies between adjacent ribs from the tips of the transverse processes posteriorly (where it communicates with the paravertebral space) to the costal cartilages anteriorly. It is bounded by intercostal muscle and membrane, the intercostalis intima muscle and parietal pleura, and the inferior surface of the rib. The external intercostal muscle is analogous to the external oblique muscle of the abdomen and extends from the tubercles to the ribs posteriorly to the costal cartilages, by which time it has thinned out to become the anterior intercostal membrane. The internal intercostal muscle runs in the same direction as the internal oblique muscle of the abdomen and extends from the sternum anteriorly to the angle of the rib where it is replaced by the posterior intercostal membrane. Deep to the intercostal space lie the innermost intercostal muscles which are relatively flimsy structures easily penetrated by local anaesthetics and the pleura. The depth of the intercostal space is greatest at the angle of the rib where it averages 8 mm. The word 'space' is really a misnomer since it is largely filled by fat, and contains from above downward the main intercostal vein, artery and nerve although anatomical variations are common.[2]

The subcostal nerve also contributes, with the first lumbar ventral ramus, to the iliohypogastric and ilioinguinal nerves which have a similar course and distribution. After leaving the vertebral column they pass inferolaterally through psoas major before piercing the transversus abdominis and running forwards in the abdominal wall superior to the iliac crest. Apart from the muscles of the abdominal wall the iliohypogastric nerve supplies the skin and fascia of the upper gluteal region and the anterior abdominal wall immediately superior to the pubis. The ilioinguinal nerve, after leaving the transversus abdominis, pierces the internal oblique muscle to enter the inguinal canal and reaches the skin through the superficial inguinal ring and the spermatic cord. It supplies abdominal wall muscles as well as skin and fascia over the pubic symphysis, the superomedial part of the femoral triangle, the anterior surface of the scrotum and root and dorsum of the penis or the mons pubis and labium majus (Fig. 8.2).

The genitofemoral nerve is closely associated with these nerves and is formed from elements of the ventral rami of L1 and L2. It descends on the anterior surface of psoas major dividing into two branches as it approaches the inguinal ligament. The genital branch goes through the deep inguinal ring into the inguinal canal from which it eventually emerges to supply the skin of the scrotum or labium majus and the adjacent part of the thigh. The femoral branch enters the thigh deep to the inguinal ligament to supply an area of skin and fascia over the femoral triangle lateral to that supplied by the ilioinguinal nerve.

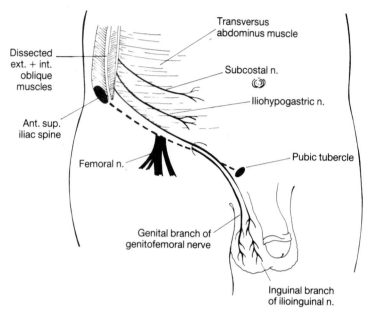

Figure 8.2 Nerves of the inguinal region.

General technique

All injections should be carried out using an aseptic technique. When only a single injection is being performed it may be possible to accomplish this without draping the patient but for catheterization techniques it is essential to guard against accidental catheter contamination during the procedure and this can only be ensured by towelling the area and wearing sterile gloves.

Some anaesthetists find it useful to prescribe opioid premedication if the block is to be performed preoperatively but in most cases a benzodiazepine will suffice. Local anaesthetics such as 0.5% lignocaine can be used for the skin and subcutaneous tissues and will do much to ensure the patient's comfort. Most patients are happy to undergo such procedures before operation when it is explained that it will provide analgesia postoperatively.

Paravertebral block

This technique was first described in 1919 but has not become popular for use in the thoracic region because of the risk of complications such as pneumothorax and central spread of local anaesthetic.

Technique

If the block is performed preoperatively the patient should lie in the prone position so that the landmarks are easily palpated. If carried out in the immediate postoperative period it is easier to use the lateral position with the operative side uppermost. By drawing the upper arm forward access to the vertebral area is increased by displacement of the subcutaneous tissues. To locate a particular vertebra it is essential to start from a fixed point, e.g. spinous process of L4 or T1, and to count from that.

Because of the downward angle of the spinous processes in the thorax it is necessary to locate the tip of the fifth spinous process to inject the sixth thoracic nerve. However this angle gradually decreases in magnitude so that at T12 the tip of the spinous process lies midway between the transverse processes of T12 and L1. A line is drawn through the superior edge of the spinous process and extended laterally 3 cm from the midline. This marks the projection of the transverse process on the skin. If a needle is inserted too medially to this point it may contact the lamina of the vertebra resulting in an injection into the spinal canal. If it is too lateral it may contact the rib leading to injection into the pleura. Careful aspiration for blood or CSF should always precede any injection.

Having determined which nerves need to be blocked the skin should be marked because the landmarks may be obscured when the area is cleaned and draped. After infiltrating the skin with local anaesthetic a 10 cm needle (e.g. 22G spinal needle) is advanced perpendicularly through the skin onto the transverse process which is usually at a depth of 2–3 cm (but may be over 6 cm in the obese patient). The needle is withdrawn slightly, inclined in a cephalad direction and advanced a further 2 cm. At this stage the needle should be passing through the superior costotransverse ligament into loose areolar tissue and it is possible to elicit a loss of resistance to injection of saline or air.[3] After negative aspiration for blood and CSF 5 ml of local anaesthetic is injected slowly. Because of its proximity, the sympathetic ganglion will also be blocked. A Tuohy needle can also be inserted in the same manner.[4] After entering the paravertebral space and with the bevel facing lateral to avoid direct epidural placement, an endhole catheter is inserted approximately 2 cm. To prevent catheter dislodgement as the patient moves it must be secured adequately with a sterile dressing. Finally, a filter is attached.

This technique is especially valuable at thoracotomy because the position of the needle can be checked while the chest is open. This is achieved by inserting the Tuohy needle during the operation itself and then asking the surgeon to inspect the paravertebral area from the inside. Once the needle is in place, 10 ml of saline is injected and if the tip is in the correct position a subpleural swelling will be visible. After successful needle placement the catheter is inserted.

The pattern of spread of local anaesthetic in paravertebral blockade is extremely variable. A single injection of 5 ml of 0.5% bupivacaine will block an average of four dermatomes, but the range is from zero to ten. When extensive block follows paravertebral injection, spread appears to be mainly into the epidural space and in some cases bilateral dermatomal block is produced. The extent of the block may also be affected by posture so that more extensive caudal spread will occur if the patient is semi-erect during injection.[5] Since the range of spread is so great, only 5 ml increments or less should be injected through a catheter. Infusions of 0.25% bupivacaine 3–10 ml/hour have been effective after thoracotomy and have been associated with less hypotension than epidural infusion.

Applications

Because of the complications associated with this technique and its unpredictable spread it should be used only for unilateral analgesia e.g. after thoracotomy, cholecystectomy through a subcostal incision, or for fractured ribs. It will provide more extensive analgesia than intercostal injections because of block of both the sympathetic supply and the dorsal primary ramus. After thoracotomy it may be necessary to insert one catheter one space above the incision and a second at a level appropriate to the drain sites. There would appear to be no benefit whatsoever in performing bilateral paravertebral block because it is simpler and quicker to insert an epidural catheter.

For postoperative analgesia 0.25% bupivacaine with 1:200,000 adrenaline to decrease absorption is recommended and should be given incrementally or by infusion as noted above. Since the risks of drug toxicity, hypotension and pneumothorax exist, careful monitoring is required and ideally the blood pressure, pulse and respiratory rates should be measured every half-hour by nursing staff who know the symptoms, signs and management of these complications. Intravenous access must be maintained and all necessary resuscitation equipment must be readily available.

Complications

The specific complications of this technique are:
Pneumothorax   The exact incidence is difficult to estimate, but may be as

high as 20 per cent, although few of these require chest drains. It is also possible that interpleural injection occurs regularly, but is unrecognized.

Epidural spread   This may be the cause of the widespread analgesia or hypotension sometimes seen.

Hypotension   This is due to sympathetic blockade, is much less common than with epidural block and should be managed along the same lines with vasopressors and intravenous fluids.

Intradural injection   If the needle is angled medially during insertion it may enter a dural sleeve. When the local anaesthetic is injected a high spinal block will result. The ensuing hypotension and apnoea will respond to conventional therapy.

Intercostal blockade

Intercostal block was first performed in 1912 and has rightly remained popular since then. The advent of long-acting drugs and catheter techniques will ensure its continuation.

Needle technique

If the block is performed preoperatively the patient should lie in the prone position. It is important to palpate the ribs carefully and this will be found to be easiest at the angle. For abdominal surgery it is sufficient to block the lower six nerves and it will not be necessary to mark them, but if in any doubt, and especially if other areas of analgesia are desired, then the ribs should be marked prior to cleaning. The angle of the rib is the preferred point of injection because the intercostal space is widest and the lateral cutaneous branch of the nerve will also be blocked.[6]

Prior to commencing the block a 20 ml syringe containing 0.5% bupivacaine with 1:200,000 adrenaline should be prepared. A 3.6 cm 22G short bevel hypodermic needle will suffice for all but the most obese patient. With the left forefinger palpating the lower border of the rib and simultaneously pushing the skin and subcutaneous tissues cephalad, the needle is inserted at right angles to the skin and down onto the bone. After making contact the needle is walked inferiorly off the rib as the left forefinger allows the skin to slide down. The needle is advanced 4 mm into the space before being anchored in position by the thumb and forefinger of the left hand. After a negative aspiration test for air and blood 3 ml of 0.5% bupivacaine with adrenaline is injected. With experience lower volumes will also produce a successful block and can be used where there is anxiety regarding toxicity. Before withdrawing the needle the left forefinger moves up to the next rib and identifies the angle so that no space is overlooked.

Controversy exists over the extent of spread of the local anaesthetic after injection[7, 8] but clinically, injections are usually limited to one space.

The intercostal nerve is a typical mixed nerve containing motor as well as sensory nerves and the author has had success in locating it using a nerve stimulator. As the needle attached to the negative electrode is advanced towards the nerve the anterior abdominal wall is inspected for rythmic twitching. It is important to ignore contractions of the intercostal muscles themselves as this may be due to local stimulation. The needle is slowly advanced and when contractions are seen the current is reduced to approximately 0.5 mA. If the contractions are maintained the needle is close to the nerve and the local anaesthetic can be injected, producing an immediate relaxation of the muscles. This method is more awkward to use in the awake patient as they tend to hold the abdominal muscles in some degree of tension making visualization of twitches difficult.

To provide analgesia after thoracotomy the block can be performed during the operation by the surgeon using the interthoracic route. Under direct vision the needle is inserted into the intercostal space close to the nerve and 2–3 ml of local anaesthetic injected into each interspace.

Applications

Intercostal blockade can be used for all of the thoracic nerves although the angles may become difficult to palpate from the sixth rib upward due to the overlying scapula, and the arm must be abducted to improve access. For postoperative analgesia it is essential to block all the dermatomes covered by an incision plus one above and below. For a midline incision bilateral injections will be required but unilateral block will suffice for a procedure such as Kocher's incision for cholecystectomy. Intercostal block of T10, 11 and 12 on the right has also been found effective for pain relief after appendicectomy.[9]

The recommended solution is 0.5% bupivacaine with adrenaline 1:200,000 because of its long duration of action. After a single injection the duration of analgesia may be influenced by the concomitant use of opioids[10] but dermatomal block lasts approximately eight hours. In order to maintain adequate analgesia it will be necessary to repeat the blocks at intervals of six to eight hours. By doing this the injections are performed before the skin sensitivity returns to normal and the procedure should not be too uncomfortable. Obviously this technique of repeated injections is extremely demanding.

Complications

Pneumothorax   The incidence of this complication decreases with experience and in some series is as low as 0.075%. Until the individual anaesthetist is fully conversant with the technique he should perform only unilateral injections in the postoperative period rather than before operations because nitrous oxide will increase any pneumothorax.

Toxicity   Blood concentrations of local anaesthetics are higher after intercostal block than any other and peak within 10 to 15 minutes. Adrenaline should always be added to the local anaesthetic solution because of this potential for producing a toxic reaction. In children doses of bupivacaine 4 mgkg^{-1} with adrenaline have produced blood concentrations below the toxic level but it is important to remain cautious and vigilant.[11] Patients must be monitored closely for 30 minutes after injection and all resuscitative equipment kept close at hand.

Intradural injection   This has been described and would appear to be a greater problem when the block is performed by a surgeon using the intrathoracic method. At thoracotomy the surgeon can see the intercostal nerve clearly and if a cuff of dura mater extends into the intercostal space the injection may be made into it. Since a percutaneus injection will be less accurately placed this complication should be much less likely.

Intercostal catheterization

In 1980 Nunn and Slavin reported that a single intercostal injection of 3 ml India ink spread subpleurally from one intercostal space to another in cadavers.[2] Despite difficulty in reproducing this finding clinically, it became apparent that injection of much larger volumes could produce widespread block.[12] Using direct visualization techniques and computerized axial tomography (CAT)[13, 14] it was apparent that spread could occur medially to the paravertebral space and then up and down to those adjacent. In some cases local anaesthetic even spread under the prevertebral fascia to the contralateral aspect of the vertebral body producing a bilateral block.

Technique

With the patient lying in the lateral position the angle of the rib is palpated. Under aseptic conditions a 16 gauge Tuohy needle is walked down off the rib as in the standard technique. With the bevel facing medially it is advanced 4 mm into the space. There have been reports of a loss of resistance as the needle penetrates the posterior intercostal membrane and a glass syringe may be used for this purpose. With the stylet removed 10 ml of saline must be injected to open up the space which is filled with fat, vessels and nerves. An end-hole catheter is then advanced a distance of 3 to 4 cm into the space. After careful removal of the needle the catheter is secured to the patient and a filter attached.

This is not an easy technique and in the author's hands (subsequently verified at thoracotomy) the failure rate is over 20 per cent, with some catheters lying superficially in the muscle layer and others in the pleural cavity itself. The injection of 20 ml of local anaesthetic produces a block of two to five dermatomes and is typically one segment above the site of insertion and one to three below. Modifications of this technique have included positioning of the catheter in the intercostal space by the surgeon before closing the chest and this should increase the success rate.

Applications

Intercostal catheters can be used in any clinical situation in which individual intercostal injections are indicated. However it must be remembered that the dermatomal spread achieved may be limited and so two catheters should be used for an extensive unilateral incision. A midline incision may require up to four catheters and this is an unattractive proposition given the high failure rate of insertion and the need for large doses of local anaesthetic.

Intercostal catheters should therefore be restricted to unilateral incisions and rib fractures. Injections of 0.5% bupivacaine with adrenaline will produce analgesia similar in duration to conventional intercostal block. Continuous infusions are theoretically possible, but have not yet been evaluated.

Complications

Toxicity   The pharmacokinetic profile is similar to that for single intercostal injection and peak blood concentrations are produced within 20 minutes. Because of the large dose of drug injected all standard precautions must be taken.

Pneumothorax   Although a large needle is required the risk of pneumothorax does not seem to be any greater than with the single injection technique in experienced hands.

Interpleural injection   It is likely that many of the papers published about intercostal catheterization have in fact been describing interpleural injection. A catheter inadvertently inserted into the pleural cavity will produce significant analgesia.

Interpleural catheterization

In 1984 it was discovered that anaesthetic placed in the pleural cavity can produce a significant effect on intercostal nerves.[15] The local anaesthetic appears to diffuse through the parietal pleura and intercostalis intima muscle to reach the intercostal nerves.[16] The sympathetic chain and phrenic nerves are also separated from the drug by only the pleura and may be similarly affected.

Technique

This block is best performed at the end of surgery because of the risk of pneumothorax. The patient is placed in the lateral position with the operative side uppermost as for intercostal block and the area around the angle of the eighth rib is cleaned and draped. To minimize the risk of lung damage the patient should be hyperventilated, remain paralysed and thus apnoeic when the needle punctures the parietal pleura. A 16G epidural needle with the bevel facing medially is advanced at an angle of 45 degrees (to lessen the risk of the sharp leading edge lacerating the visceral pleura) through the skin and down onto the angle of the rib. It is then 'walked' over the top of the rib and into the seventh interspace so avoiding the intercostal vessels and nerves which usually lie in the superior part of the space. At this stage the stylet is removed and a device for detecting negative interpleural pressure is attached. This could be a well lubricated glass syringe or, the author's choice, a Macintosh balloon.

A loss of resistance is often noted as the needle tip pierces the posterior intercostal membrane. The needle is advanced slowly until it enters the pleural cavity when the Macintosh balloon deflates. It is often necessary to advance the needle another few millimetres so that all of the bevel lies within the pleural space or it may be difficult to insert the catheter. The Macintosh balloon is removed and the catheter is inserted through the needle quickly. Great care must be taken to avoid the entry of a significant amount of air. If the tip of the needle is in the correct tissue plane there should be virtually no resistance to catheter insertion and five centimetres can be advanced rapidly into the space. After this the needle is withdrawn over the catheter leaving the latter in place. A syringe is attached and aspirated: a little air is frequently removed but more importantly a few millilitres of serous fluid are often aspirated and this is consistent with correct placement of the catheter. It is now secured to the patient and a filter is attached securely.

The most important indicators of correct catheter placement are the signs of negative interpleural pressure, the ease with which the catheter can be inserted through the Tuohy needle and the aspiration of serous fluid. 20 ml of 0.5% bupivacaine with 1:200,000 adrenaline is then injected over three to four minutes to allow the detection of an accidental i.v. injection. A reduction in wound pain is usually seen within five minutes and reaches a maximum at thirty minutes.[17, 18] The duration of effect depends on the concentration of bupivacaine and a 0.5% solution with adrenaline will last approximately six hours. The extent of the block is strongly influenced by gravity.[18] If a block of the upper thoracic dermatomes is required the patient should lie head down for fifteen minutes after injection. Since the lower edge of the lung reaches the tenth rib during normal tidal excursions it may be possible to insert the catheter below this level to decrease the probability of lung damage. Gravity may then be used to help achieve the appropriate block – however this approach has not been evaluated.

In the supine patient CAT scan has demonstrated that an interpleural injection of 20 ml of local anaesthetic and contrast mixture can spread along the full length of the paravertebral gutter.[19] The block is rarely as dense as that from conventional intercostal injections and there may be little objective evidence of its presence. Sympathetic block appears to be common and upper thoracic block can produce Horner's syndrome and a rise in temperature of the ipsilateral limb.

Applications

Interpleural catheterization has been used widely for analgesia after unilateral operations such a cholecystectomy by subcostal incision, nephrectomy and mastectomy. Pain after unilateral fractured ribs and thoracotomy can also be well controlled, but the chest drain must be clamped for at least ten minutes after injection so that the local anaesthetic drug is not drained away.[20]

Bilateral interpleural catheters have been used to control pain from midline incisions but should be used with great caution. There is the risk of bilateral pneumothorax and also a significant risk of toxicity because 20 ml of 0.5% bupivacaine is injected into each side.

In order to gain the maximum benefit with the lowest risk of toxicity, the duration of pain relief should be established after the first dose and then repeat injections made at appropriate intervals. Continuous infusion of 0.25% bupivacaine at a rate of 8 ml/hr provides good analgesia after cholecystectomy.

Complications

Pneumothorax   Despite the apparent risk involved in placing a catheter in the pleural cavity the incidence of major pheumothorax requiring a chest drain is low provided the technique is not used in patients with previous history of chest surgery, pleurisy, pneumonia or severe emphysema. When chest X-rays have been taken routinely, small pneumothoraces have been detected in up to 30 per cent of patients. Air can often be aspirated from the catheter immediately after insertion but the volume is usually small. Even if catheter insertion has been uneventful a high index of suspicion should be maintained and erect inspiratory and expiratory chest X-rays taken if a significant pneumothorax is suspected.

Toxicity   Blood concentrations peak twenty minutes after injection. Large doses of bupivacaine have been used without obvious systemic effect, but adrenaline should always be included to decrease the rate of absorption.[21] There has been a report of a convulsion in a patient with a history of recent pneumonia who was given 150 mg bupivacaine. Pleural inflammation may lead to an increase in the rate of absorption of local anaesthetic and is another reason for not using the technique in patients with recent pulmonary infection.

Ilioinguinal, iliohypogastric and genitofemoral blocks

These nerves innervate the inguinal and femoral region, an area in which many operations are carried out. Judicious use of nerve blocks will provide good postoperative analgesia, with little need for additional drugs.

Technique

Since the operations may obscure tissue planes and the presence of dressings make palpation difficult, these blocks are best performed after induction of anaesthesia and before surgery. A 20 ml syringe filled with 0.5% or 0.25% bupivacaine with adrenaline is prepared and a 22G needle, preferably with a short bevel, is attached. The first stage is to block the ilioinguinal and iliohypogastric nerves.

The anterior superior iliac spine is palpated, and the skin around it and the inguinal region is cleaned. The needle is inserted perpendicularly through the skin 2–3 cm medial and inferior to the spine. If the needle is advanced carefully it is possible to appreciate the change in resistance as it goes through the subcutaneous fat and then reaches the aponeurosis of the external oblique muscle. When the needle is scraped superficially over the surface of the aponeurosis it has a distinctive 'feel'. The needle is advanced a further 3–4 mm through the aponeurosis and a 'click' can usually be felt. 8 ml of the solution is injected and as the needle is withdrawn 2–3 ml is deposited in the subcutaneous tissue.

The next stage is to block the genitofemoral nerve. The injection site is 2 cm superior to the midpoint of the inguinal ligament. The syringe and needle are advanced to lie again on the aponeurosis of the external oblique. The needle is advanced a little further until the 'click' is felt and 5 ml of solution injected.

The third stage requires an injection to block those pain fibres which cross the midline. 5 ml is injected subcutaneously from the pubic tubercle to a point midway to the umbilicus. This technique produces analgesia for up to twelve hours.

To provide continuous analgesia it is possible to perform an 'inguinal catheterization'. After the ilioinguinal and iliohypogastric injection a 16G Tuohy needle is inserted down through the aponeurosis of the external oblique. An end-hole epidural catheter is then inserted through the needle into the tissue plane between the aponeurosis and the internal oblique muscle. Usually only 2–3 cm of catheter can be introduced. Since this is done preoperatively the surgeon can check the tissue plane in which the catheter is lying during the operation. If the catheter is misplaced it is most often found in the substance of the internal oblique and the surgeon can probe with a finger up towards the anterior iliac spine and hook the catheter down into the correct plane. When it appears that the initial injection of local anaesthetic is wearing off a top-up of 20 ml of 0.25% bupivacaine with adrenaline is given. This produces analgesia for up to eight hours and can be repeated easily.

Applications

The 'single injection' technique is most suited to inguinal and femoral hernia repair. It produces good postoperative analgesia and permits a lighter level of general anaesthesia with better quality recovery. Block of the genitofemoral nerve frequently produces a 'bupivacainoma' in the surgical field and the surgeon should be warned of this preoperatively.

Inguinal catheterization has only been used to prolong analgesia after hernia repair, but may have a place in providing analgesia for other procedures in this region of the body, e.g. Caesarean section by Pfanensteil incision.

Complications

Bowel perforation   This is only a risk during the genitofemoral block and does not appear to be a major problem. However this stage of the block should be omitted if there is incarcerated or strangulated bowel in the hernia.

Toxicity   Provided that safe doses are given and adrenaline is used, toxicity should not be a major problem even in children.

Summary

Traditional intercostal block remains a popular technique for producing perioperative analgesia, but it is distressing for the patient to have it repeated. Unfortunately intercostal catheterization has not lived up to its early promise as a useful method of prolonging conventional intercostal blockade. The incidence of complications associated with paravertebral block is high, but the technique may be particularly valuable after thoracic surgery. Interpleural catheterization appears to be an effective technique for providing unilateral analgesia and will gain in popularity if it proves to be safe as well as effective. For prolonged bilateral analgesia with minimal risk of complications epidural infusion remains the technique of choice after abdominal surgery.

References

1. Purcell-Jones G., Pither C. E., Justins D. M. Paravertebral Somatic Nerve Block: a clinical, radiographic and computed tomographic study in chronic pain patients. *Anesth. Analg.* 1989; **68**: 32–9.
2. Nunn J. F., Slavin G. Posterior intercostal nerve block for pain relief after Cholecystectomy. *Brit. J. Anaesth.* 1980; **52**: 253–9.
3. Eason M. J., Wyatt R. Paravertebral thoracic block – a reappraisal. *Anaesthesia* 1979; **34**: 638–42.
4. Conacher I. D., Korri M. Postoperative paravertebral blocks for thoracic surgery. *Brit. J. Anaesth.* 1987; **59**: 155–61.
5. Mathews P. J. Govenden V. Comparison of continuous paravertebral and extredural infusion of bupivacaine for pain relief after thoracotomy. *Brit. J. Anaesth.* 1989; **62**: 204–5.
6. Moore D. C., Bush W. H., Scurlock J. E. Intercostal nerve block: a roentgenographic anatomic study of technique and absorption in humans. *Aneasth. Analg.* 1980 **59**: 815–25.
7. Moore D. C. Intercostal nerve block: spread of india ink injected to the rib's costal groove. *Brit. J. Anaesth.* 1981; **53**: 325–9.
8. Mowbray A., Wong K. K. S. Low volume intercostal injection. A comparative study in patients and cadavers. *Anaesthesia* 1988; **43**: 633–4.
9. Bunting P., McGeachie J. F. Intercostal nerve blockade producing analgesia after appendicectomy *Brit. J. Anaesth.* 1988; **61**: 169–72.
10. Mcquay H. J., Carroll D., Moore R. A. Post-operative orthopaedic pain – the effect of opiate premedication and local anaesthetic blocks. *Pain* 1988; **33**: 291–5.
11. Rothstein P., Arthur R., Feldman H. S., Kopf G. S., Covino B. G. Bupivacaine for intercostal nerve blocks in children: blood concentrations and pharmacokinetics. *Anesth. Analg.* 1986; **65**: 625–32.
12. Murphy D. F. Continuous intercostal nerve blockade. *Brit. J. Anaesth.* 1984; **56**: 627–9.
13. Mowbray A., Wong K. K. S., Murray J. M. Intercostal catheterisation. *Anaesthesia* 1987; **42**: 958–61.
14. Kuhlman G., Ahmad R., Cauquil P., Roche A., Edouard A. Bilateral analgesia after unilateral intercostal block. *Anesthesiology.* 1987, **67**: 3A 284.
15. Kvalheim L., Reiestad F. Interpleural catheter in the management of postoperative pain. *Anesthesiology.* 1984; **61**: A231.
16. Vadeboncouer T. R., Pelligrino D. A., Riegler F. X., Albrecht R. F. Interpleural bupivacaine in the dog: distribution of effect and influence of injectate volume. *Anesth. Analg.* 1989; **68**: S301.

17.   Stromskag K. E., Reiestad F., Holmqvist E. W. O., Ogenstad S.
Interpleural administration of 0.25%, 0.375% and 0.5% bupivacaine
with epinephrine after cholecystectomy. *Anesth. Analg.* 1988; **67**: 430–4.
18.   McIlvaine W. B., Knox R. F., Fennessey P. V., Goldstein M. Continuous
infusion of bupivacaine via interpleural catheter for analgesia after thoracotomy in children. *Anesthesiology* 1988; **69**: 261–4.
19.   Brismar B., Petterson N., Tokics A., Strandberg A., Hedenstierna G.
Postoperative analgesia with interpleural administration of bupivacaine –
adrenaline. *Acta Anaesth. Scand.* 1987; **31**: 515–20.
20.   Rosenberg P. H., Scheinin BM-A., Lepantalo M. J., Lindfors O.
Continuous intrapleural infusion of bupivacaine for analgesia after
thoracotomy. *Anesthesiology* 1987; **67**: 811–3.
21.   El-Naggar M. A., Raad C., Yogaratnam G., Poritz A., Bennet B.
Interpleural intercostal nerve block using 0.75% bupivacaine. *Anesthesiology* 1987; **67**: A258.

9

Regional techniques for postoperative analgesia of the limbs

H. B. J. Fischer
B. E. Smith

General considerations

Few opportunities exist for the anaesthetist to provide postoperative analgesia of 12–36 hours duration unless a catheter technique is used. However, such a duration of analgesia can be readily achieved in both the upper and the lower limb, by a single dose of a concentrated solution of a long-acting local anaesthetic agent, placed in close proximity to the nerve trunks. Although a nerve stimulator is neither essential nor a substitute for a thorough knowledge of relevant surface and neuroanatomy it can be a major asset in performing many peripheral blocks,[1] particularly in the obese or where the anatomy is abnormal.

There are a number of questions that the anaesthetist must ask of him/herself, the patient and the surgeon before selecting any particular technique:

1   Is it appropriate to use a technique that may leave the limb devoid of all feeling and possible movement for up to 36 hours? Some patients find these effects even more distressing than postoperative pain, and a full discussion of this aspect is advisable.

2   Is there likely to be much pain after surgery? The patient may complain bitterly about a limb that is anaesthetic for most of the day if his previous experience had indicated that there would be minimal discomfort.

3   Will surgery be confined to just one area? There is little point in providing analgesia in one limb if there are other sources of pain which will require systemic narcotics.

4   Would the patient prefer to be asleep during surgery? There is a tendency to categorize patients as needing either a general *or* a regional anaesthetic. In fact the two modalities are complementary, not mutually

exclusive. A decision by the patient to be unaware during surgery should not condemn him to suffer its painful consequences.

5   Will surgery be confined to the upper or lower part of the limb? This is an important distinction because, as a general rule, the more peripheral the site of the block, the longer the duration of analgesia that may be produced and the less the extent of motor blockade.

6   Will a tourniquet be used during surgery? If so, the analgesia must be extensive enough to block tourniquet pain secondary to pressure and the resulting ischaemia.

7   How long might surgery take? With a long-acting agent such as bupivacaine there should not be any problem in producing a block that extends well into the postoperative period. However, the fear of delayed onset might influence the clinician to use a more rapidly acting agent and to sacrifice the postoperative benefit. With careful selection of techniques this sacrifice need not be made.

8   Would an extended period of sympathetic blockade be advantageous? This is particularly important in cases of crush injury or in vascular reconstructive surgery. The maintenance of good peripheral 'run-off' may influence the outcome of vascular reconstructions or the eventual degree of function of a severely injured limb.[2]

Postoperative mobilization

It is important to warn the patient and his attendants that motor blockade may outlast sensory blockade. A limb that feels normal will not necessarily function properly, and all patients who have received a peripheral block must be mobilized with caution. This is obviously important after lower limb blocks, but the role of the upper limb in both balance and protection from injury should not be forgotten.

Ischaemic pain

The overzealous application of compression dressings, plaster casts or splints can lead to peripheral vascular insufficiency. One of the cardinal symptoms in this situation is pain. It is imperative that the patient's attendants are experienced in the effects of regional anaesthesia, and know that the limb should be checked regularly for other evidence of impaired circulation.

Patient positioning

The medical and nursing staff must ensure that the limbs are positioned in a way that will not produce complications from pressure effects or hyperextension of joints. The limb should be well padded by the judicious use of pillows, and the legs positioned to avoid calf compression which may predispose to deep vein thrombosis.

Nerve block technique

Many standard texts provide descriptions of plexus and discrete nerve blocks for the upper and lower limb and it is not our intention to restate these here. In most texts the methods described are of blocks used in isolation to provide anaesthesia for surgery, and they do not consider either postoperative analgesia, or the patient undergoing surgery with superimposed general anaesthesia. In the authors' practice 80 per cent of patients receive some form of regional anaesthetic technique, but in only 32 per cent is surgery performed under regional anaesthesia alone. Such combined general and regional anaesthetic techniques require that additional factors are taken into account when planning the anaesthetic.

Use of vasoconstrictors

Most authors quote recommended volumes and concentrations of local anaesthetic agents. The majority specify the use of adrenaline-containing solutions, particularly with lignocaine, to allow the use of more concentrated solutions of larger volumes. The duration of the block appears to be a secondary consideration. If halothane is to be given during surgery then the use of adrenaline may be contraindicated. In this situation, the use of alternative vasoconstrictors should be considered.[3]

Speed of onset/duration of action

To some extent the speed of onset of a regional anaesthetic technique is inversely related to its duration of action. The speed of onset and the duration of action of an individual drug can be improved by increasing the concentration used. Certainly for sciatic nerve block a low volume/high concentration solution may give better clinical results than a high volume/low concentration of the same mass of drug.[4] The problem of slow onset is further reduced if a general anaesthetic is to be administered. In this situation, the duration of action of the local anaesthetic is the principal determinant of selection.

Choice of local anaesthetic agent

In the discussions that follow, bupivacaine is usually recommended because it is assumed that the duration of postoperative analgesia should be as long as possible. This is not always the case, and shorter acting agents such as prilocaine or lignocaine may be used to provide more transient effects.

Upper limb techniques

As a general rule, optimal postoperative analgesia of the upper limb is seldom achieved by a single injection and the best results may be obtained by a combination of nerve blocks using more than one agent.[5]

Surgery of the shoulder

There are a number of regional techniques that may provide good analgesia after shoulder surgery.

Cervical paravertebral block   The skin overlying the shoulder joint receives its nerve supply from the supraclavicular nerves and the lateral cutaneous nerve of the arm (C3, 4 and 5). The sole somatic supply to the shoulder joint and its surrounding structures is the suprascapular nerve (predominantly C5, although a minor contribution may be made by C4). Paravertebral block of C3-C5 with bupivacaine 0.5% will thus produce effective postoperative analgesia. Two to four millilitres may be injected in each paravertebral space, although the full dose can be given by a single injection because longitudinal spread will occur (Fig. 9.1).

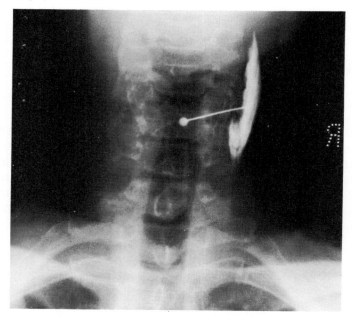

Figure 9.1   Cervical paravertebral injection: 7ml of bupivacaine mixed with 3ml of Niopan 300 have been injected at the C4/5 level. The solution is seen to spread from C2 above to C6 below.

The latency of the block is usually of the order of 10 minutes although more rapid onset is relatively common. The duration of action is typically 8–12 hours in adults, but may be up to 18 hours in the elderly. Paralysis of the phrenic nerve on the blocked side must be almost invariable, but this does not appear to produce any problem in practice, even in patients with marked respiratory disease. It would seem prudent, however, to avoid bilateral blocks. A degree of sympathetic blockade to the head is common and is also of little significance, although the patient should be warned of its likely occurrence.

Interscalene block   This approach to the brachial plexus is probably the most widely used regional technique for surgery of the shoulder. Unfortunately, as many clinicians have found, the block is not always adequate as the sole anaesthetic technique. The usual reasons for this are either inadequate blockade of the supraclavicular nerves or the C7, C8 and T1 dermatomes, the anterior aspects being more of a problem in this regard than the posterior.

However, the technique has much to commend it when combined with light general anaesthesia. A suitable local anaesthetic agent is bupivacaine 0.25%–0.5% without adrenaline in a volume of 30–40 ml depending upon the status of the patient. Whilst the use of up to 200 mg of bupivacaine may at first sight seem excessive, this dose is unlikely to cause systemic toxicity provided that it is deposited in the correct site in a young healthy adult.[6] The addition of adrenaline will delay absorption, but it has been shown that the dose contained in 40 ml of a 1:200,000 solution can produce significant cardiovascular disturbance.[3]

The authors have used such doses routinely in adult males for several years and have yet to see any significant adverse effect. With this dosage, the onset is usually less than 10 minutes and the duration of action 8–16 hours.

Supraclavicular brachial plexus block   This approach can be effective in shoulder surgery when an anterior approach to the joint is used, e.g. the Putti-platt operation. Its principal drawback is a significant incidence of failure to block the suprascapular nerve, but if this is blocked separately then good results are usually achieved. The results can be further improved by turning the patient onto the unblocked side after injection to improve the central spread of the solution. The total dosage used is as for interscalene block, but with 5 ml of bupivacaine 0.5% for the suprascapular block. The latency of the block appears to be somewhat shorter, and the duration longer, than with interscalene block.

Suprascapular nerve block   This nerve provides all the somatic innervation of the shoulder joint and its surrounding structures. Most of the pain experienced by patients after surgery of the shoulder joint appears to result from deep structures rather than from the skin. When surgery is performed under general anaesthesia the addition of a suprascapular block can provide considerable postoperative analgesia, especially when combined with sub-cutaneous infiltration of the skin incision. Although suprascapular nerve block is generally performed by the posterior approach, the anterior can also be used. In thinner patients, in whom the coracoid process is readily palpable, the anterior approach is the easier of the two. It is also more easily performed at the end of surgery, because the patient may remain supine rather than be turned to the lateral or semi-sitting position, as is normally required for the posterior approach.

The agent of choice is either 0.5% or 0.75% bupivacaine 3–8 ml. For skin infiltration, bupivacaine 0.25% with adrenaline is used. Onset is approximately 10 minutes and duration 12–18 hours with the 0.5% solution and up to 30 hours with 0.75%.

Surgery of the arm

With the exception of intravenous regional anaesthesia (Bier's block), the most common regional anaesthetic technique used for upper limb surgery is brachial plexus block. When considering postoperative analgesia this is not the best choice because 80 per cent of all upper limb surgery is performed distal to the elbow. The majority of patients fall into one of four categories:

1. Surgery proximal to or on the elbow – tourniquet required.
2. Surgery proximal to or on the elbow – tourniquet not required.
3. Surgery distal to the elbow – tourniquet required.
4. Surgery distal to the elbow – tourniquet not required.

In the first two categories brachial plexus block alone is the method of choice. In general, the more proximal the surgery, the more proximal should be the site of injection, and interscalene, subclavian perivascular and supraclavicular blocks are all appropriate. If prolonged postoperative analgesia is required the drug of choice is bupivacaine 0.5%, in a volume of 30–40 ml in the adult. It is curious that whilst in theory it should be necessary to block the intercostobrachial nerve (from T2) when using a tourniquet, this is rarely needed in practice.

For surgery distal to the elbow which requires a tourniquet the anaes-thetist must consider two opposing factors. Firstly the duration of wound analgesia should generally be as along as possible, but the duration of accompanying unwanted motor block of the shoulder, upper arm and elbow should be as short as possible. It is both unnecessary and undesirable to produce complete motor block of the limb if only the hand has been operated upon. In this category the best results are obtained by using bupivacaine for peripheral blocks of the median, ulnar and radial nerves at either the elbow or the wrist. The tourniquet pain may be obtunded with a light general anaesthetic or with a brachial plexus block using a shorter acting agent such as prilocaine. Using this combination, motor block of the upper arm will persist for little more than two hours, whilst distal analgesia may persist for 12–24 hours.[5] This is particularly important in day case anaesthesia where the patient should regain control of the arm as soon as possible after surgery, but should not require narcotic analgesics which could delay discharge.

For surgery distal to the elbow when a tourniquet is not required there is no indication for brachial plexus block as a means of providing postoperative analgesia. Distal nerve blockade is the method of choice.

Median nerve block   This nerve can be blocked at the level of either the elbow or the wrist and the drug of choice depends on the duration of analgesia required. Latency should have little influence on selection because the onset of the block is rapid whichever agent is employed. With 0.75% bupivacaine the duration of action is in the order of 12–18 hours in most patients; 3–5 ml of solution is sufficient whichever drug is used.

Radial nerve block   The radial nerve may be blocked at 3 sites: 8 cm above the lateral epicondyle; at the level of the epicondyle; or where it emerges from beneath the brachioradialis muscle 8–10 cm proximal to the wrist. Subcutaneous infiltration on the dorsum of the wrist from the ulnar to the radial styloid will block the branches supplying the dorsum of the hand and fingers. Blockade at the elbow will almost invariably be accompanied by block of the lateral cutaneous nerve of the forearm, a useful point to remember for surgery on the forearm. For blocks performed at, or proximal to, the elbow, 5 ml of plain bupivacaine 0.5% or 0.75% should be used and will generally provide postoperative analgesia for 12–18 hours. At the wrist 10 ml is usually required, and 0.25–0.5% solution should be used. The duration of action is noticeably shorter with this method, but up to 12 hours analgesia may be expected.

Ulnar nerve block   The ulnar nerve can be blocked 2–3 cm proximal to the ulnar groove at the elbow or 2–4 cm proximal to the ulnar styloid at the wrist. For the latter the authors favour a medial approach to the nerve, rather than the more traditional anterior approach because it produces more reliable blockade of the dorsal branch. From 2 to 5 ml of either 0.75% or 0.5% bupivacaine provides postoperative analgesia for 12 to 18 hours.

Influence of tourniquet ischaemia   If a tourniquet is applied proximal to the point of peripheral nerve blockade shortly after injection of the local anaesthetic solution, there is evidence that the duration of analgesia is extended in the almost total absence of circulation.[5] Little of the local anaesthetic is cleared from the site of injection and this will result in greater intraneural concentration. The higher the peak value concentration, the longer the duration of action.[4]

Digital nerve block   The digital nerves (two dorsal and two palmar) can be blocked at the level of either the metacarpals (interosseous block) or classically at the base of the finger. The interosseous method may be less painful in the conscious patient and may have a marginally shorter latency. In both cases, 4–6 ml of solution is required for each digit and the concentration of solution injected will depend upon the number of digits to be blocked. If this is more than two then a more proximal block should be considered. When bupivacaine 0.5% is used, the duration of postoperative analgesia is generally 6–12 hours.

Solutions containing adrenaline should not be used in this situation.

Intravenous regional anaesthesia   This technique enjoys considerable popularity, particularly for outpatient surgery. The drug of choice is prilocaine 0.5% without adrenaline because of its low systemic toxicity. Unfortunately, the duration of analgesia after tourniquet release is seldom prolonged. In cases where surgery is expected to cause significant postoperative pain Bier's block is a poor choice unless augmented by discrete nerve blocks as discussed above.

Lower limb techniques

With the increased use of regional anaesthesia to provide postoperative analgesia, a marked difference has developed between the methods used for upper and lower limbs. Whereas plexus and individual nerve blocks are routine in the upper limb, epidural block is seldom used, but the reverse is true in the lower limb. Epidural and spinal techniques are used almost to the exclusion of other methods, despite the widespread bilateral block which affects autonomic, bladder and bowel function. The immobility that such central blocks produce may also be a disadvantage.

This disparity of approach may reflect current teaching of regional anaesthetic techniques and also the relative inaccessibility of the lumbo-sacral plexus. However a single peripheral block may produce up to 36 hours of high quality analgesia without the adverse effects of a more central technique and with minimal impairment of mobility.

Four nerves, the sciatic, femoral, obturator and lateral cutaneous nerve of the thigh arise from the lumbo-sacral plexus to supply the leg. Knowledge of the distribution of the terminal branches of the femoral and sciatic nerves is important when providing analgesia of the lower leg and foot. As with the upper limb, it is not adequate to base the selection of nerve blocks solely on the site of skin incision, for the innervation of deep structures must also be considered. This is well illustrated in surgery of the knee where the incision may be confined to the femoral nerve territory, but the joint itself is supplied by all four nerves.

Surgery of the hip

Analgesia for surgery of the hip is most easily produced by spinal or epidural block. This does not mean that it necessarily produces the best results in all cases, and other techniques may be considered, particularly when spinal anaesthesia is contraindicated.

Psoas compartment block A single injection technique for lumbar plexus block has been described[7] and relies upon identification of the fascial sheath that surrounds the psoas major. The lumbar plexus lies within this space and may be blocked by the injection of up to 50 ml of bupivacaine 0.25%. This may produce analgesia for up to eight hours. There is debate as to whether the block is a true compartment block or, in effect, merely lumbar paravertebral block.

Inguinal paravascular ('3 in 1') block This approach was first described by Winnie in 1973.[8] It is similar to the psoas compartment block in that the principal branches of the lumbar plexus are anaesthetized within the neurovascular bundle. The standard approach to the femoral nerve is used, but a volume of up to 30 ml is injected to encourage proximal spread. Digital pressure distal to the point of injection may aid this. Studies using contrast media would suggest that such volumes are not always necessary, and as little as 10–15 ml will be adequate in most cases. When bupivacaine 0.75% is used, analgesia may persist for 36 hours.

With this approach the femoral and obturator nerves are usually blocked, but the lateral cutaneous nerve of the thigh, which leaves the bundle more proximally, may be missed and require a separate injection. It is our impression that the success rate of the technique decreases as patient age increases. This may reflect partial obliteration of the space through which the local anaesthetic must spread. In such cases, discrete block of the individual nerves may produce better results.

Blockade of the lumbar plexus and its nerves will only produce partial analgesia for hip surgery. The skin overlying the greater trochanter is supplied by the subcostal nerve, while the hip joint itself receives fibres from the sciatic nerve. These nerves must be blocked separately if full surgical anaesthesia and total postoperative analgesia are required.[9]

Surgery below the hip

For all other procedures on the lower limb separate blockade of the appropriate nerves produces a better result than plexus block, particularly where it is necessary to restrict the volume of local anaesthetic used. The femoral nerve may be effectively blocked with 5–8 ml of bupivacaine 0.75%, the obturator with 2–5 ml, the sciatic with 3–6 ml and the lateral cutaneous nerve with 5–8 ml. A total volume of 25 ml may produce complete analgesia of the leg for up to 48 hours, yet have minimal effect on autonomic function, and none on the bowel, bladder or the other limb. The more accurate the needle placement, the smaller the volume of anaesthetic solution required, and the shorter the latency of the block.[4] The use of a peripheral nerve stimulator is considered necessary for such accuracy.[10]

Use of tourniquet

As in the upper limb the use of a tourniquet must be borne in mind when planning the local anaesthetic regimen. If general anaesthesia is to be administered then tourniquet pain poses no problems, but in other cases it will be necessary to block all four major nerves. In this situation the use of a shorter acting agent is appropriate for all the nerves except those that supply the operative site. This will reduce unwanted postoperative effects in other nerve territories, but maintain the duration of analgesia.

Surgery of the knee

Because the knee joint is supplied by branches of all four major nerves, many clinicians opt for central neural blockade as the simplest way of providing anaesthesia and postoperative analgesia.[11] However, major peripheral nerve block will produce much more prolonged analgesia from a single injection and this is particularly useful after joint replacement surgery which may require early vigorous mobilization. Anaesthetists regularly involved with such procedures find it a useful technique. Where early mobility is required, as in day case arthroscopic surgery which is likely to cause only modest or transient postoperative pain, discrete nerve blocks or intra-articular block are more appropriate.

Femoral nerve   Although the femoral nerve is relatively superficial and generally thought to bear a constant relationship to the femoral artery, it can be difficult to block. Emerging from beneath the inguinal ligament the nerve may have already divided into its anterior and posterior divisions or even their respective branches. It may be located more medially than usual, lying either deep or superficial to the femoral artery making localization difficult and possibly painful in the conscious subject.

It is important to identify accurately the posterior division because this ultimately supplies the knee joint (and gives origin to the saphenous nerve). The distribution of paraesthesiae may be misleading because they may be produced by stimulation of the anterior division or one of its branches. Again, a peripheral nerve stimulator may be useful in this situation by producing pulse-synchronous contractions in the quadriceps muscle which derives its motor supply from the posterior division.

If bupivacaine 0.5% is used the latency is usually 10–15 minutes and duration 24–36 hours. With prilocaine 1% without adrenaline, onset is more rapid and the duration 2–6 hours.

Obturator nerve   This nerve is generally regarded as being difficult to block.[11] Using the classical, anatomically-based techniques this is true, but with the inferior approach using a nerve stimulator,[12] a success rate in excess of 90 per cent is readily achieved. The anterior division supplies a small, variable area of skin over the supra-medial aspect of the knee. As with the femoral nerve it is important to identify the posterior division which supplies the adductor muscles and the knee joint. The use of a nerve stimulator to produce pulse-synchronous contractions of the adductor muscles greatly improves accuracy. Onset of block is generally more rapid than with the femoral nerve for any given agent, although duration of action is similar.

Lateral cutaneous nerve of the thigh   This is an important, but often neglected nerve. It is often blocked if the thigh is to be the donor site for skin grafts, but its importance in knee surgery is frequently overlooked. It supplies the knee joint through the patellar plexus and must be blocked if total anaesthesia of the knee is required. If a nerve stimulator is used to locate this purely sensory nerve in the conscious patient, paraesthesiae must be -evoked, so its value is limited. Latency and duration of action are similar to femoral nerve block.

Sciatic nerve   The sciatic nerve is distributed predominantly to the back of the thigh, the lower leg and foot, but it does have an important articular branch which supplies the posterior capsule of the knee and the posterior horns of the menisci. The nerve may be blocked where it emerges from the sciatic notch using the posterior approach,[13] or more distally using the anterior,[14] supine posterior[15] or lateral[16] approaches. Whichever method is used, a nerve stimulator is needed for a high success rate.

The sciatic is essentially double-barrelled consisting of both tibial and common peroneal components running together. In some cases the two nerves arise separately from the sacral plexus and run a parallel, but separate, course through the thigh. More often it divides into two sections high in the thigh rather than in the popliteal fossa. It is imperative to identify and block both components particularly when using a high concentration low volume technique.

With bupivacaine 0.5% latency of block can be surprisingly protracted (1 hour in many cases) but, by way of compensation, the duration of action often exceeds 36 hours. If a much shorter latency is required, prilocaine 3 or 4% with vasoconstrictor has a latency of 10–15 minutes, but still provides analgesia for up to 12 hours.[4]

Intra-articular block Routine diagnostic arthroscopy and many intra-articular procedures can be performed in the conscious patient using an intra-articular block. This can provide remarkable postoperative analgesia if bupivacaine is used. The 0.25% solution is infiltrated at the instrument entry sites, and the 0.5% solution injected into the joint cavity. Up to 40 ml may be used because most of the solution is removed during arthroscopy. It is vital, however, to ensure that the drug is deposited within the knee joint and not into the surrounding structures or blood vessels. Provided that the solution remains within the joint cavity for more than 15 minutes, analgesia will persist for 6–12 hours. A major advantage of this technique is that the knee joint is stable, there is no associated motor deficit and patients can literally walk unaided from the operating table, without pain.

Surgery of the lower leg

Below the knee joint, all somatic innervation is derived from the sciatic or saphenous nerves and both are readily blocked at the knee. Thus postoperative analgesia for all forms of surgery below the knee can be produced without the more widespread motor and sensory effects that follow more proximal sciatic and femoral block.

Popliteal block The sciatic nerve usually divides at the apex of the popliteal fossa into its two principal branches, the common peroneal and tibial nerves. As mentioned earlier, the level of division is variable and it is again advisable to identify both components by seeking parasthesiae or muscle stimulation in both distributions. A volume of 5–10 ml is required and results in analgesia for up to 36 hours with bupivacaine 0.5%.

Saphenous nerve The saphenous nerve is the terminal branch of the femoral and supplies the medial side of the lower leg from the knee to the medial malleolus. It is closely related to the long saphenous vein so great care must be taken to avoid intravascular injection. At knee level there is seldom much subcutaneous tissue and the block is little more than a subcutaneous infiltration. Relatively dilute solutions of local anaesthetic agents can be used and bupivacaine 0.25% can be expected to produce analgesia within 10 minutes and last for 12–24 hours.

Surgery of the foot

Most of the foot is supplied by terminal branches of the sciatic nerve, and the saphenous may innervate part of the medial aspect. Good postoperative analgesia may be achieved by blocking these branches at ankle level. With practice, ankle blocks can be very successful and the posterior tibial nerve, which supplies the whole of the weight-bearing surface of the foot, is almost invariably blocked if up to 5 ml of solution is used.

Full ankle block requires about 20 ml of local anaesthetic solution, but not all five nerves need to be blocked for a particular operation. The smaller volume required permits the use of relatively concentrated solutions and bupivacaine 0.75% will produce analgesia which persists for more than 36 hours. Such a duration can be a source of alarm to both surgeon and anaesthetist, who may fear that nerve injury has occurred. It is essential that all involved including the patient, are aware of this long duration.

Because of the close relationship of the deeper nerves to the arteries supplying the foot, it is wise to avoid injections at this level in patients with circulatory insufficiency.

Vascular surgery of the leg

Although the sciatic and femoral nerves are predominantly somatic, both are accompanied by sympathetic fibres. Blockade of both nerves results in a degree of vasodilatation similar to that produced by lumbar sympathectomy. This can be of value in both diagnosis and therapy of peripheral vascular disease. In vascular surgery sympathetic blockade increases graft blood flow and may reduce the incidence of occlusion. The surface temperature of the blocked limb is increased and it may be that the increased blood flow may promote healing after debridement or amputation.

Continuous techniques

While percutaneous catheter techniques are used in central neural blockade, they are seldom used in peripheral blocks. There are many reasons for this, particularly that central blocks tend to have relatively short durations, but such techniques may also be used for limb blocks when indicated. In the upper limb, continuous brachial plexus block via the supraclavicular,[17] subclavian perivascular[18] and the axillary route[19] are all relatively simple. The authors favour a Seldinger type technique for the more proximal methods, and the direct insertion of an intravenous cannula for the axillary approach.

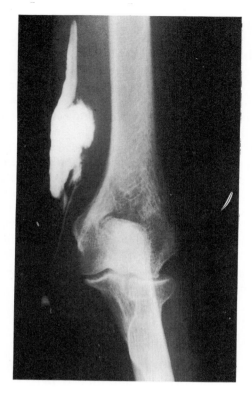

Figure 9.2   Percutaneous catheterization of the median nerve: 3ml of bupivacaine mixed with 2ml of Ultravist 300 has been injected through the catheter. The spread of solution along the neurovascular space is clearly seen.

Percutaneous cannulation of more peripheral nerves in the upper limb is difficult, although the median nerve in the antecubital fossa is an exception (Fig. 9.2). However, the indications for continuous block of these nerves are fortunately few, and brachial plexus block generally offers a more suitable alternative.

In the lower limb, continuous blockade is indicated more commonly, and both the femoral[20] and sciatic[21] nerves lend themselves to such techniques (Fig. 9.3). In both cases the Seldinger technique is preferred, and is particularly easy in the case of the femoral nerve. Continuous blockade of one or both nerves has been employed for postoperative analgesia, chronic pain relief, treatment of sympathetic dystrophy and peripheral vascular disease. Continuous neural blockade is valuable in diabetic patients with peripheral ischaemia and ulceration. Not only is the pain relieved, but control of blood sugar and ketoacidosis is markedly improved. The avoidance of narcotic analgesics in such patients can result in a marked improvement in cooperation and a reduction in nausea, vomiting and constipation. As a result, it is usually possible to restore

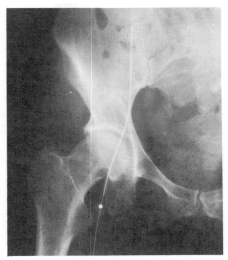

Figure 9.3   Femoral and sciatic catheterization. Fig. 9.3(a) above shows a 16-gauge catheter (Secalon Seldy) inserted alongside the femoral nerve. Fig. 9.3(b) over shows both femoral and sciatic catheters in place. In both cases, 6ml of local anaesthetic mixed with 4ml of Omnipaque has been injected through the catheters. A – spread of solution around the psoas muscle. B – solution flowing through the sciatic notch to the sacral plexus. C – entry point for sciatic catheter. D – entry point for femoral catheter.

a reasonable degree of dietary control, which greatly facilitates insulin administration.

The placement of percutaneous catheters not only permits the anaesthetist to prolong the block, but also allows extension, intermittent use, or the sequential use of different agents as the clinical situation changes. A brachial plexus block could, for example, be induced with prilocaine 2% for a rapid onset for surgery, and then be maintained with bupivacaine for prolonged surgery or postoperative analgesia.

Phantom limb pain

In the early period after limb amputation, up to 90 per cent of patients will experience phantom limb symptoms.[23] Only a proportion of them will suffer true pain, the majority experiencing some degree of dysaesthesia or dyskinaesthesia. Many reports have suggested that phantom limb pain is more likely to occur in patients who have had pain prior to amputation.[23–25] There is also evidence to suggest that the nature of the phantom pain tends to be similar in quality, severity and location to the preoperative pain.[24, 25] Preliminary clinical studies suggest that central blockade reduces the incidence of phantom pain when used preoperatively.[26] Presumably major peripheral blocks would have the same effects. It is not known if regional

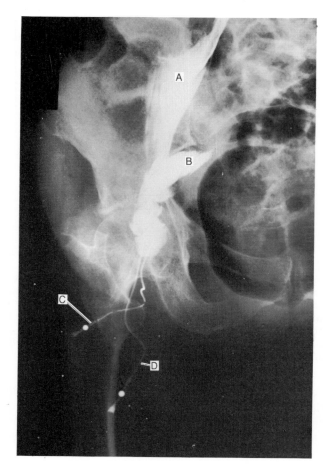

Figure 9.3(b)

blockade used only at the time of surgery has a significant effect on the incidence of phantom pain. Further studies are in progress to assess this.

The influence of opioids

The effectiveness of analgesia in continuous nerve blocks may be increased by the additional administration of an opioid (Chapter 7). The use of opioids in spinal and epidural blockade is now commonplace, and the efficacy of such techniques are well documented. More recently, opioids have been injected close to peripheral nerves with some success.[27] Injection of fentanyl 25 µg into the lumbo-sacral plexus resulted in significant analgesia of several hours duration and was not associated with any change in motor, autonomic or other sensory modality.[28]

The mode of action of opioids in this situation is far from clear, but a number of mechanisms have been suggested.[28] These include systemic absorption, axoplasmic transport to the spinal cord and a direct effect on nerve conduction. Fentanyl is a weak local anaesthetic and is made up in a hypotonic solution so that an osmotic effect cannot be excluded.[29] It is probably wiser to inject only isotonic solutions close to nerves because of the risk of neurolysis.

Conclusion

Ideally, when using regional anaesthetic techniques for postoperative analgesia they should abolish pain to a degree, and for a time, that obviates the need for any other form of analgesia. After most minor or intermediate surgery such a goal is relatively easy to achieve. After major surgery, complete abolition of pain is often possible, but only at an unacceptably high cost in terms of adverse effects, delay in patient mobilization, or man-hours spent managing the patient. Perhaps a secondary end point is appropriate for such patients. The immediate, severe postoperative pain is obtunded by the regional technique for long enough to allow analgesia to be continued effectively with other methods. This approach is usually far more practicable, and is often as popular with patients as it is with hospital staff.

References

1. Smith B. E. The distribution of evoked paraesthesiae and effectiveness of brachial plexus block. *Anaesthesia* 1986; **41**: 1112–5.
2. Cousins M. J., Wright C. J. Graft, muscle, skin blood flow after epidural block in vascular surgical procedures. *Surg. Gynaecol. Obstet.* 1971; **133**: 59–64.
3. Kennedy W. F., Bonica J. J., Ward R. J. *et al.* Cardiovascular effects of epinephrine when used in regional anaesthesia. *Acta Anaesth. Scand.* 1966; **23**: 320–33.
4. Smith B. E., Siggins D. High concentration low volume block of the sciatic nerve. *Anaesthesia* 1988; **43**: 8–11.
5. Smith B. E., Challands J. F., Suchak M., Siggins D. Regional anaesthesia for upper limb surgery – a technique of combined brachial plexus and discrete nerve blocks. *Anaesthesia* 1989; **44**: in press.
6. Arthur G. R., Wildsmith J. A. W., Tucker G. T. Pharmacology of local anaesthetic drugs. In: Wildsmith J. A. W., Armitage E. N. (eds); *Principles and Practice of Regional Anaesthesia*. Edinburgh, Churchill-Livingstone, 1986.
7. Chayen D., Nathan H., Chayen M. The psoas compartment block. *Anesthesiology* 1976, **45**: 95–9.
8. Winnie A. P., Rammamurthy S., Durrani A. The inguinal paravascular

technic of lumbar plexus anesthesia; the '3 in 1' block. *Anesth. Analg.* 1973; **52**: 989–96.

9.   Smith B. E., Allison A. Nerve block for hip surgery. *Anaesthesia* 1987; **42**: 1016–7.

10. Smith B. E., Allison A. Use of a low-power nerve stimulator during sciatic block. *Anaesthesia* 1987; **42**: 296–8.

11. Macrae W. A. Lower limb blocks. in: Wildsmith J. A. W., Armitage E. B. (eds); *Principles and Practices of Regional Anaesthesia*. Edinburgh, Churchill-Livingstone, 1987.

12. Smith B. E., Fischer H. B. J. A simplified approach to obturator nerve block. *Regional Anaesthesia* 1989: In press.

13. Labat G. *Regional Anesthesia: its Technic and Clinical Applications*. Philadelphia, W. B. Saunders, 1924.

14. Englesson S. Nerve Block in the Region of the Hip-Joint. In: Eriksson E. (ed); *Illustrated Handbook in Local Anaesthesia, 2nd edn*. London, Lloyd-Luke, 1979.

15. Raj P. P., Parks R. L., Watson T. D., Jenkins M. T. New single position supine approach to sciatic-femoral nerve block. *Anesth. Analg.* 1975; **54**: 489–93.

16. Guardini R., Waldron B. A. , Wallace W. A. Sciatic nerve block: a lateral approach. *Acta Anaesth. Scand.* 1985; **29**: 515–9.

17. Hemel V., Van Fuick M., Baumgartner E. A longitudinal supraclavicular approach to the brachial plexus for the insertion of plastic cannulas. *Anesth. Analg.* 1981; **60**: 352–5.

18. Rosenblatt R. M., Vress J. C. Modified Seldinger technique for continuous brachial plexus block. A new approach. *Anesthesiology* 1979; **51**: 565–6.

19. Selander D. Catheter technique in axillary plexus block. Presentation of a new method. *Acta Anaesth. Scand.* 1977; **21**: 324–9.

20. Rosenblatt R. M. Continuous femoral anaesthesia for lower extremity surgery. *Anesthesia and analgesia* 1980; **59**: 631–2.

21. Smith B. E., Fischer H. B. J., Scott P. V. Continuous sciatic nerve block. *Anaesthesia* 1984; 39; 155–7.

22. Jensen T. S., Rasmussen P. Amputation. In: Wall P. D., Melzack R. (eds), *Textbook of Pain*. Edinburgh, Churchill-Livingstone, 1985.

23. Mitchell S. W. Injuries of nerves and their consequences. Philadelphia, J. B. Lippencott, 1872.

24. Riddoch G. Phantom limbs and body shape. *Brain* 1941; **64**: 197–222.

25. Parkes C. M. Factors determining the persistance of phantom pain in the amputee. *J. Psychosomatic Res.* 1973; **17**: 97–108.

26. Bach S., Noreng M. F., Tjelldeu N. U. Phantom limb pain in amputees during the first 12 months following limb amputation after preoperative lumbar epidural blockade. *Pain* 1988; **33 (3)**: 297–301.

27. Sanchez R., Neilsen H., Heslet L., Iversen A. D. Neuronal blockade with morphine – a hypothesis. *Anaesthesia* 1984; **39**: 788–9.

28. Smith B. E., Pinnock C., Fischer H. B. J., Trotter T., Scott P. V. Unilateral analgesia following injection of fentanul into the lumbosacral plexus. *Lancet* 1987; **1**: 1497.

29. Power I., Brown D. T., Wildsmith J. A. W. Effect of fentanyl on nerve conduction. *Brit. J. Anaesth.* 1988; **61**: 507.

10

Principles of patient management

J. H. McClure

Regional anaesthesia is once again being commonly used[1] as part of a 'balanced' anaesthetic technique.[2, 3] In 1913 Crile[2] described his kinetic theory of shock after surgery in which he suggested that during surgery the central nervous system (CNS) was still exposed to traumatic impulses which were not excluded by inhalational anaesthesia alone. Anoci-association, which he defined as the exclusion of these impulses from the CNS was only attained by the combination of cocaine used peripherally and the concurrent use of inhalational anaesthesia. Recent work[4] supports the hypothesis that neural blockade established before surgery may reduce postoperative pain long after the direct effect of the local anaesthetic has worn off. Sequential analgesia is achieved by administering systematic analgesics before the complete regression of conduction blockade and avoids the sudden appreciation of pain.[5]

Evidence that the use of regional anaesthesia reduces surgical morbidity[6] is fully discussed in Chapter 4 and the superior quality of analgesia provided by conduction blockade has also been discussed in previous chapters. It is not the intention here to discuss further the management of individual techniques, but to offer general guidelines in the safe establishment of these techniques into routine clinical practice.

On humanitarian grounds, pain prevention is more appropriate than pain relief.[7] Good pain relief or pain prevention is stated to be achievable, at a price. Just what is the cost? Is this measured in terms of increased workload or utilization of scarce resources or even reduced patient safety? Our speciality is now beginning to assess the acceptance, efficiency and safety of techniques of conduction blockade and selective spinal analgesia in clinical practice. There has been little published on the widespread use of the techniques though a nationwide survey in Sweden[8] suggests that selective spinal analgesia is widely used. It appears that the improved quality of analgesia offered by these techniques has resulted in their rapid introduction into clinical practice.[9] But what should be the constraints?

Most regional anaesthetic techniques have recognized side-effects and complication. The choice of such a technique should always be weighed-up against the side-effects and risks of conventional or on-demand intramuscular opioid analgesia. Intramuscular opioid analgesia is generally considered safe provided major restraints are applied in prescribing and administration. Nursing and surgical staff must be aware of the benefits of providing patients with better analgesia and this requires a considerable amount of education, particularly in the initial stages of instituting change in routine. Once the benefits have been observed in improving overall patient management without putting the patients at risk, it is not difficult to maintain motivation for these techniques provided supervision is maintained at senior level. Most regional anaesthetic techniques do not have major implications in terms of workload or resource with the exception of continuous central neural blockade and selective spinal analgesia.[10]

Patient management may be conveniently divided into three components.

Preoperative visit

The majority of patients have little experience of surgery and most expect postoperative pain. Expectations of pain relief are realistically low. A recent assessment of patients' satisfaction with postoperative pain relief showed that for 70 per cent of patients the pain was at least as bad as they had expected.[11] Children and their parents also deserve explanation, particularly if the loss of sensation following a conduction block is likely to be misinterpreted by a young child as absence of a limb or other appendage! In the interest of safety many anaesthetists will only perform major peripheral or central neural blocks on conscious cooperative patients[12] and this should also be discussed with the patient preoperatively. Motor dysfunction, loss of proprioception or urinary retention, which may be evident postoperatively, should also be explained. Bladder catheterization may be routine if central neural blockade or selective spinal analgesia is used. It is advisable to discuss this with the surgeon, particularly if there is a perceived risk of bacteraemia at catheterization. The possible occurrence of other side-effects such as pruritus or nausea should also be discussed if they occur frequently.

The availability of the appropriate level of nursing care and monitoring equipment for the postoperative period should also be determined at this stage if this is not routinely provided. The out-patient requires further consideration of his or her ability to travel home. The avoidance of parenteral opioid analgesia should ensure street-fitness, but care must be taken to ensure that complete function has returned. If out-patients are to be discharged from hospital with a residual nerve block they and their attendants need to be warned to avoid accidental injury.

Anaesthesia

Premedication providing a calm and cooperative patient is advisable particularly if a regional block is performed before the induction of general anaesthesia. Parenteral opioids should be avoided if bolus administration of spinal opioids is planned.[13] Central neural blocks and brachial plexus blocks are generally performed in the awake and cooperative patient. Regional anaesthesia in children, some lower limb blocks, caudal blocks, intercostal, interpleural and paravertebral blocks are generally performed after the induction of general anaesthesia or at the end of surgery.

Techniques of peripheral nerve blockade can usefully be performed during general anaesthesia in children using a nerve stimulator.[14] The axillary approach to the brachial plexus is recommended in children due to the greater risk of pneumothorax in the supraclavicular approach because of the softer cartilaginous first rib.[15] A dose of 0.5 ml.kg^{-1} bupivacaine provides useful postoperative analgesia after upper limb surgery. Single dose epidural analgesia via the caudal route is commonly used in children after induction of general anaesthesia for surgery to the lower limbs, ano-perineal or genito urinary and abdominal surgery below the umbilicus.[16] Caudal blocks with 0.25% bupivacaine provide between 4 and 8 hours of good analgesia and Armitage's dosage regimen for children is easy to use.[17]

An epidural block should be sited at the appropriate level to allow the desired segmental analgesia without resorting to large volumes of local anaesthetic to achieve spread.[18] It is essential that a good and efficacious segmental block is achieved by bolus dose of local anaesthetic before a continuous epidural infusion is commenced in the postoperative period. The appropriate drugs, solutions, pumps and other equipment should be prepared during surgery if an epidural infusion is planned. The unavailability of commericially-produced large volume dilute local anaesthetics requires the preparation of solutions from ampoules in solutions and equipment generally used for intravenous infusion. Herein lies a hazard of inappropriate connection and administration of local anaesthetic intravenously, and careful labelling is required.

Postoperative care

Out-patients require separate consideration as different end-points of return of function and lack of sedation are intended. The use of techniques such as intravenous regional anaesthesia and intra-articular local anaesthesia of the knee with short-acting local anaesthetics should allow early discharge from hospital. The combination of light general anaesthesia, particularly when a tourniquet is used for limb surgery, with distal peripheral nerve blocks is preferable to plexus blocks to avoid major dysfunction of the limb. The prescription of oral analgesia for the out-patient is advisable if pain is anticipated once neural blockade wears off. Out-patients should be reviewed on the understanding that full function of a limb, for example, has returned before discharge. Nerve blocks with the potential for late onset of a complication, e.g. pneumothorax following supraclavicular brachial plexus block, should be avoided in out-patients. Resident surgical staff should know what to expect in terms of duration of a block and who to contact if they require advice. Simple peripheral blocks may be of great benefit should opioid analgesia be unsuitable, particularly in children undergoing day-care surgery. Ilioinguinal and iliohypogastric nerve blocks are useful following orchidopexy and herniotomy[19] and wound infiltration with local anaesthetic gives comparable analgesia to caudal block.[20] Topical application of local anaesthetic gel, or block of the dorsal nerve of the penis provide good analgesia after circumcision.[21, 22] It is interesting that simple infiltration or the topical application of local anaesthetics in some circumstances provides comparable analgesia to more central blocks without the risk of significant side-effects or complication.

Peripheral nerve blocks

Nursing staff should know the expected duration of effect of peripheral nerve blocks and should be encouraged to give prescribed analgesia before the local anaesthetic block has regressed completely. Such sequential analgesia[5] is beneficial following most in-patient surgery and avoids sudden awareness of pain when a continuous catheter technique is used. Care should be taken to avoid pressure sores following a single dose technique with a long-acting local anaesthetic or a catheter technique. Sudden movement of anaesthetic joints should be avoided particularly in the arthritic patient. Plaster of Paris casts may cause pressure ischaemia, and feet and hands should be observed for circulatory insufficiency because pain, one cardinal sign of ischaemia, has been blocked.

Regional blockade of the thorax, including paravertebral, intercostal and interpleural blocks, share the complications of pneumothorax and systemic local anaesthetic toxicity. Both are rare, but may present late, and resident surgical staff and nursing staff should be aware of the symptoms and signs of these complications. There should be no doubt about treatment of such complications and who is available should such a complication occur. It is suggested that analgesia charts are used[23] to assess the adequacy of analgesia together with the normal recordings of temperature and cardiovascular and respiratory measurement. A simple visual analogue score would be better than no score at all and would provide some feedback which is lacking in everyday practice. The reverse side of such a chart could contain details of possible complications, their presentation and their management. The use of catheter techniques requires close supervision by the responsible anaesthetist. The use of interpleural infusions of bupivacaine has been described in Chapter 8: it has also been used successfully in children, providing effective analgesia following anterior spinal fusion or repair of aortic coarctation.[24]

Central nerve blocks

The benefit of even short periods of epidural blockade in the postoperative period has been observed after cholecystectomy.[25] Maintenance of seg-mental blockade for 12 hours postoperatively by low thoracic epidural administration of local anaesthetic using a bolus top-up technique pro-vided superior analgesia to parenteral opioid by intermittent intramuscular injection or intravenous infusion. A decreased incidence of pulmonary complication and chest infection was also observed, and was presumed to be due to good analgesia provided by the epidural block which did not restrict the patients' ability or desire to breath deeply or cough in the immediate postoperative period thus reducing small airway closure and atelectasis.

The continuous infusion of local anaesthetic using a catheter, particularly in the lumbar and thoracic epidural space, allows the extension of analgesia well into the postoperative period. Maintenance of sympathetic blockade may be beneficial in terms of lower limb blood flow and control of blood pressure particularly after reconstructive vascular surgery. Provided the tip of the epidural catheter is sited close to the nerve roots transmitting pain, excellent analgesia may be achieved with a small dose of local anaesthetic given continuously by volumetric pump. An occasional top-up may be required should the block recede or become unilateral. This would appear to be necessary less frequently than in obstetric practice in labour when the sensory input is progressively changing. The equipment required to safely administer local anaesthesia by infusion is fully described in Chapter 7. Regular changes in position of the patient are recommended to avoid pressure ischaemia and to reduce the incidence of unilateral block.

Intermittent top-ups are an alternative means of maintaining a continuous block in the postoperative period but have the following disadvantages:

1. they do not provide a continuous block and painful intervals are common;[18]
2. they require frequent medical intervention;
3. they cause haemodynamic instability and the patient requires very close supervision after each top-up.

This is not an efficient means of providing pain relief and rarely achieves pain prevention. A pump delivering small intermittent top-ups has been described[26] but has not gained widespread acceptance.

When using an epidural infusion consideration should also be given to pain arising outwith areas covered by the epidural block, and parenteral opioids should be prescribed in addition when necessary. Respiratory depression should not normally occur with a continuous infusion of local anaesthetic alone unless the catheter is inadvertently placed intrathecally resulting in a gradual progression of spinal block,[27] or an overdose of parenteral opioid is given in addition. Sympathetic block, however, may cause hypotension which should be treated according to clinical need. Generally treatment is indicated if the patient is symptomatic or is elderly when hypotension is less well tolerated. Patients with any degree of hypovolaemia do not tolerate sympathetic blockade. The former should be considered the most likely cause of hypotension in the postoperative patient. In the absence of central venous pressure monitoring, poor peripheral perfusion in the upper limbs in the absence of hypothermia is a good clinical indicator of hypovolaemia. Possible continuing haemorrhage should be considered and fluid therapy is indicated. Hypotension in a vasodilated patient requires therapy with a vasoconstrictor. Ephedrine and methoxamine should be available in the surgical ward and resident medical staff should know when and how to use these drugs.

The masking of the symptoms and signs of intrathoracic, intra-abdominal or pelvic haemorrhage is often quoted as a major disadvantage of maintenance of an epidural block in the postoperative period. Provided attendant surgical staff are aware that haemorrhage may occur and do not attribute all hypotension to the epidural block then the guidelines above are appropriate. Indeed, the loss of sympathetic reflex activity allows earlier detection of continuing blood loss because of the decreased tolerance to hypovolaemia and a fall in blood pressure is quickly apparent.

Urinary retention may be problematic in the uncatheterized patient and nursing staff should be aware that this may occur and cause breakthrough pain on occasion. This would appear to be more common in the immediate period after surgery, perhaps due to intravenous fluid therapy, bladder filling during surgery and the more widespread block which is present immediately postoperatively. Other complications include nausea and vomiting, particularly when sitting up, due to hypotension secondary to sympathetic blockade. Sitting up should be discouraged, particularly in the early postoperative period, until the block has regressed to a segmental level covering the wound.

Once it is established that the patient is in a stable condition and there is no indication of complication or progressive extension of the block, it is the author's view that these patients may be nursed in a normal postoperative surgical ward. An acceptable level of nursing supervision in a general surgical ward is assumed. It is not appropriate to care for these patients in a single room without direct supervision. There must be a resident anaesthetist in the hospital who is aware of the patients undergoing epidural local anaesthetic infusion, and to whom resident surgical and nursing staff can consult. The frequency of observation of vital signs depends on the patient's clinical condition but a minimum of half-hourly pulse, blood pressure and respiration is appropriate. All nursing staff must be aware of the benefits, management and complications of epidural anaesthesia; it is essential that nursing staff unfamiliar with the technique are not asked to be responsible for such patients without supervision, particularly at night when medical staff are not so readily available.

The volume of local anaesthetic infused each hour should be recorded as a check on the function of the pump and the epidural catheter system and to reduce the risk of human error. The use of a chart to record the vital signs and volume of local anaesthetic administered has been instrumental in achieving acceptance of these techniques. The nursing staff should receive written guidelines on acceptable limits of blood pressure, heart rate and respiration on this chart and it is useful to provide brief details of the symptoms and signs of the complications which require notification to the medical staff. It has not been our practice to ask nursing staff to monitor the upper level of sensory block, but a regular assessment of motor activity in the lower limbs may be useful. A regular review by the anaesthetist allows assessment of the adequacy of analgesia and the extent of dermatomal spread to be measured.

Chest physiotherapy may be distressing and an additional bolus top-up given prior to this is appreciated by the patient and may make physiotherapy more efficient. Lumbar epidural block[28] has been used widely in children and more recently the thoracic epidural approach has been advocated.[29] Continuous epidural infusions have been used successfully after major lower limb and genito urinary surgery in children. A dose of 0.25% bupivacaine at 0.08 ml.kg.$^{-1}$ hr^{-1} has been recommended.[30]

Selective spinal analgesia

The use of epidural or intrathecal opioids provides good analgesia without sympathetic blockade in the postoperative period. The avoidance of respiratory depression seen with parenteral opioids has, however, not been obtained when opioids are selectively applied to the spinal cord. The use of morphine alone either intrathecally or epidurally has a significant incidence of late respiratory depression.[13] There is controversy regarding whether respiratory depression may be gradual or sudden in onset but it is generally accompanied by somnolence. A major deficiency is inherent during all monitoring which utilizes intermittent measurement or observation. The event did not suddenly occur but, more correctly, was suddenly noticed. Theoretically the use of more fat-soluble opioids is safer, but late respiratory depression has again been described.[31] The combination of local anaesthetic with opioid given by epidural infusion will provide better postoperative analgesia but introduces the risk of respiratory depression.[32, 33] The current level of reporting of the risk of respiratory depression with epidural opioids suggests that it is necessary to provide continuous nursing supervision for a patient who is under the influence of a spinally administered opioid. This level of supervision is not generally available in a busy surgical ward or the single room. It is currently recommended that such patients are continuously observed.

Accurate respiratory monitoring is notoriously difficult at the bedside, and at present there would appear to be no monitor available which substitutes for, or is as reliable as, continuous nursing observation. Respiratory inductance plethysmography, apnoea alarms, capnography and pulse oximetry have all been tried, but are not totally accurate in identifying either a reduction in respiratory rate or airway obstruction. Nursing supervision by the traditional measurement of respiratory rate on a half-hourly or hourly basis is a useless method of detecting respiratory depression. However, recording of vital signs, etc., on an analgesia chart is again recommended if only to make the nursing staff aware of the symptoms and signs of complications, the possibility of sudden onset and the action they are required to take. Some centres advise that naloxone is immediately to hand and the nursing staff are instructed in administering it intravenously.[34]

Epidural administration of morphine has been used for postoperative pain relief in children[35] and though there have been no reports of frank respiratory depression the ventilatory response to carbon dioxide is depressed.[36] Intrathecal opioids have not been used widely in children. The use of intrathecal morphine has been described as giving good pain relief but is associated with a high incidence of respiratory depression.[37]

Conclusions

Peripheral nerve blocks are simple to do and provide excellent analgesia which may be prolonged. Developments in disposable needle design and peripheral nerve stimulators have allowed more accurate and less traumatic localization of nerves. Neural blockade, however, must not be at the expense or loss of significant function, particularly in the ambulant patient. The use of infiltration, or even topical anaesthesia, appears to provide good analgesia after body surface or extremity surgery, with minimal side-effects. Distal discrete peripheral nerve blocks with long-acting local anaesthetics may be preferable to plexus anaesthesia, particularly in the out-patient in whom limb function should be retained.

Analgesia after surgery to body cavities presents a greater challenge. Good analgesia for both somatic and visceral pain would appear to be optimally provided by local anaesthtic and/or opioid placed centrally within the neuraxis. Central neural blockade and selective spinal analgesia with opioids, however, demand appropriate postoperative supervision. Resources may be best centralized to allow continuous nursing supervision (in Recovery or High Dependency areas) of patients who are known to benefit from these techniques. An analysis of hospital costs when epidural analgesia was provided postoperatively to high risk surgical patients determined a saving in terms of intensive care costs.[38] It is an attractive goal to be able to admit all patients undergoing major surgery to such a High Dependency area but this will require either resources or reorganization and perhaps both.

Today it is apparent that many enthusiastic clinicians manage patients postoperatively on general surgical wards with epidural infusions and intercostal and interpleural catheters. This demands a degree of attention by those individuals involved which is unattractive to many whose commitments within the operating theatre are already stretched. This is unfortunate because the provision of good postoperative pain relief, or more appropriately pain prevention, does require commitment and resources to provide it safely. There is a parallel to the development of epidural services in obstetrics in the 1950s and 60s when the need was perceived and eventually realized in most major centres in the UK. An Acute Pain Service has been achieved in obstetrics, but it has not been without problems, requiring definition of the standards necessary for its safe delivery. This has made a paper from Seattle and the accompanying Editorial in *Anesthesiology* all the more welcome.[34] The group in Seattle have developed an Anesthesiology-based postoperative pain management service. Their stated goals in implementing this acute pain service were to:

1. improve postoperative analgesia;
2. train anesthesiology residents in methods of postoperative pain management;
3. apply and advance new analgesia methods;
4. carry out clinical research in the area of postoperative pain management.

The service is provided by an attending physician, anesthesiology resident and clinical nurse specialist on a 24-hour basis. After 18 months of operation, continuing growth reflects the popularity of the service among patients and surgeons. This is an undoubted development in quality of care produced at a cost and it will be interesting to view progress in the 1990s.

Most patients anticipate postoperative pain, but few anticipate either its severity or the poor quality of relief offered by traditional parenteral opioid analgesia. Undoubtedly many feel they should not complain fearing they will be labelled demanding or weak in spirit. It is essential therefore that if regional blockade is used the patient is not suddenly exposed to pain as the block regresses. The administration of opioid and/or non-steroidal anti-inflammatory drugs will provide sequential analgesia tailored to the patient's needs and changing perception of pain.

It is within our means to prevent postoperative pain but this must not be at the expense of safety. Standards and facilities vary widely in hospital practice and it is essential that those embarking on acute pain management examine their available facilities closely to ensure that patient safety is not jeopardized.

References

1.   Smith G. Local Anaesthesia (editorial). *Brit. J. Anaesth.* 1986; **58**: 691.
2.   Crile G. W. The kinetic theory of shock and its prevention through anoci-association (shockless operation). *Lancet* 1913; **ii**: 7–16.
3.   Lundy J. S. Balanced Anaesthesia. *Minnesota Med.* 1926, **9**: 399–404.
4.   Tverskoy M., Cozacov C., Ayache M., Bradley E. L., Kissin I. Postoperative pain after inguinal herniorrhaphy with different types of anaesthesia. *Anesthesia and Analgesia* 1990; **70**: 29–35.
5.   Wildsmith J. A. W. Developments in local anaesthetic drugs and techniques for pain relief. *Brit. J. Anaesth.* 1989; **63**: 159–64.
6.   Scott N. B., Kehlet H. Regional anaesthesia and surgical morbidity. *Brit. J. Surg.* 1988; **75**: 299–304.
7.   Armitage E. N. Postoperative pain – prevention or relief. (Editorial) *Brit. J. Anaesth.* 1989; **63**: 136–8.
8.   Rawal N., Arneil S., Gustafsson L. L., Alvi R. Present state of extradural and intrathecal opioid analgesia in Sweden. A nationwide follow-up survey. *Brit. J. Anaesth.* 1987; **59**: 791–9.
9.   Bromage P. r. The price of intraspinal narcotic analgesia; basic constraints (Editorial). *Anesthesia and Analgesia* 1981; **60**: 416–3.
10.   Morgan M. The rational use of intrathecal and extradural opioids. *Brit. J. Anaesth.* 1989; **63**: 165–88.
11.   Kuhn S., Cooke K., Collins M., Jones J. M., Mucklow J. C. Perceptions of pain relief after surgery. *Brit. Med. J.* 1990; **300**: 1687–90.
12.   Bromage P. R. The control of post-thoracotomy pain. *Anaesthesia* 1989, **44**: 445.
13.   Cousins M. J., Mather L. E. Intrathecal and epidural administration of opioids. *Anesthesiology* 1984; **61**: 276–310.
14.   Yaster M., Maxwell L. G. Paediatric regional anaesthesia. *Anesthesiology* 1989; **70**: 324–38.
15.   Arthur D. S., McNicol L. R. Local anaesthetic techniques in paediatric surgery. *Brit. J. Anaesth.* 1986: **58**: 760–78.
16.   Broadman L. M., Hannallah R. S., Norden J. M., McGill W. A. 'Kiddie Candals', experience with 1154 consecutive cases without complications. *Anesthesia and Analgesia* 1987; **66**: 748–54.
17.   Armitage E. N. Caudal block in children. *Anaesthesia* 1979; **34**: 396.
18.   Green R., Dawkins C. J. M. Postoperative analgesia. The use of continuous drip epidural block. *Anaesthesia* 1966; **21**: 372–8.
19.   Shandling B., Steward D. J. Regional analgesia for postoperative pain in paediatric outpatient surgery. *J. Paed. Surg.* 1980; **15**: 477–81.
20.   Lafferty P. M., Gordon N. H., Winning R. J. A comparison of postoperative pain relief techniques in orchidpexy. *Annals R. Coll. Surg. Eng.* 1990; **72**: 7–8.

21. Tree-Trakarn T., Pirayavaraporn S. Postoperative pain relief for circumcision in children: comparison among morphine, nerve block and topical analgesia. *Anesthesiology* 1985; **62**: 519–522.

22. Soliman M. G., Tremblay N. A. Nerve block of the penis for postoperative pain relief in children. *Anesthesia and Analgesia* 1978; 495–8.

23. Mitchell R. W. D., Smith G. The control of acute postoperative pain. *Brit. J. Anaesth.* 1989; **63**: 147–58.

24. McIlvaine W. B., Knox R. F., Fennessey P. V., Goldstein M. Continuous infusion of bupivacaine via intrapleural catheters for analgesia after thoracotomy in children. *Anesthesiology* 1988; **69**: 261–4.

25. Cuschieri R. J., Morran, C. G., Howie J. C., McArdle C. S. Postoperative pain and pulmonary complications: comparison of three analgesic regimens. *Brit. J. Surg.* 1985; **72**: 495–8.

26. Scott C. B., Schweitzer S., Thorn J. Epidural block in Postoperative Pain Relief. *Reg. Anesth.* 1982; **7**: 135–9.

27. Matovskova A. Epidural Analgesia. Continuous mini-infusion of bupivacaine into the epidural space during labour. *Act Obste. Gynaecol. Scand. (suppl)* 1979; **83**: 1–52.

28. Ruston F. G. Epidural anaesthesia in infants and children. *Can. Anaesth. Soc. J.* 1954; **1**: 37–41.

29. Arthur D. S. Postoperative thoracic epidural analgesia in children. *Anaesthesiology* 1980; **35**: 1131–6.

30. Desparmet J., Meistelman C., Barre J., Saint–Maurice C. Continuous epidural infusion of bupivacaine for postoperative pain relief in children. *Anesthesiology* 1987; **67**: 108–10.

31. Brockway M. S., Noble D. W., Sharwood-Smith G. H., McClure J. H. Profound respiratory depression after extradural fentanyl. *Brit. J. Anaesth* 1990; **64**: 243–5.

32. Cullen M. L., Staren E. D., El-Ganzouri A., Logas W. G., Ivankovich A. D., Economov S. G. Continuous epidural infusion for analgesia after major abdominal operations. A randomised, prospective double-blind study. *Surg.* 1985; **98**: 718–26.

33. Lee A., Simpson D., Whitfield A., Scott D. B. Postoperative analgesia by continuous extradural infusion of bupivacaine and diamorphine. *Brit. J. Anaesth.* 1988; **60**: 845–50.

34. Ready L. B., Oden R., Chadwick H. S., Benedetti C., Rook G. A., Caplan R., Wild L. M. Development of an anaesthesiology-based postoperative pain management service. *Anesthesiology* 1988; **68**: 100–6.

35. Dalens B., Tanguy A., Haberer J. P. Lumbar epidural anaesthesia for operative and postoperative pain relief in infants and young children. *Anesthesia and Analgesia* 1986, **65**: 1069–1073.

36. Attia J., Ecoffey C., Sandovk P., Gross J. B., Samii K. Epidural morphine in children. Pharmacokinetics and carbon dioxide sensitivity. *Anesthesiology* 1986; **65**: 590–4.

37. Jones S. E. F., Beasley J. M., MacFarlane D. W. R., Davis J. M., Hall-Davies G. Intrathecal morphine for postoperative pain relief in children. *Brit. J. Anaesth.* 1984; **56**: 137–40.

38. Yeager M. P., Glass D. D., Neff R. K., Brink-Johnsen T. Epidural anesthesia and analgesia in high risk surgical patients. *Anesthesiology* 1987; **66**: 729–36.

Index